ESSENTIAL MEDICAL TERMINOLOGY

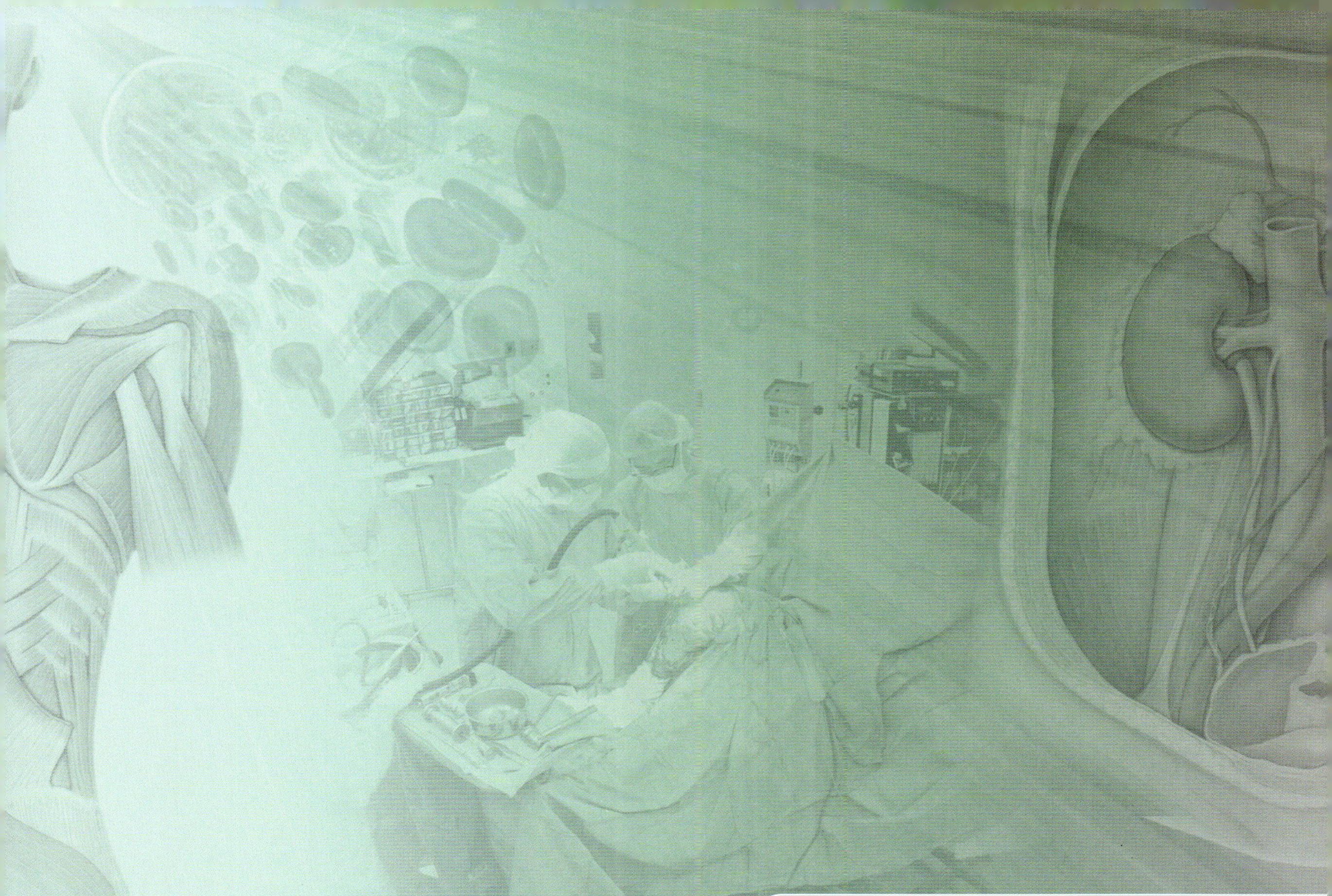

ESSENTIAL

MEDICAL TERMINOLOGY

신영순 · 김대식 · 김봉경 · 김양호 · 박상묵 · 박창은 · 심문정 · 육근돌
이영종 · 이재식 · 허성호 · 현성희 · 최원창 · 황구연 · 홍승복 · 최승구

고려의학

머리말

21세기 정보통신의 시대를 맞이하여 전 국민 의료보험에 따른 의료수요의 증가와 함께 보건의료계의 의료정보관리체계의 구축을 비롯한 의약품의 개발과 CT, MRI, 초음파 등 원격진료를 통한 의료영상의 도입으로 인하여 보건의료산업이 더욱 성장할 수 있는 촉매역할을 함으로써 의료기술이 눈부시게 발전해 가고 있다.

이러한 추세에 따라 고도로 전문화된 새로운 보건 의료 인력에 대한 수요가 급증하고 있는 실정이며, 당연히 그에 따른 교육과정에 대한 관심과 기대가 커지고 있다. 그러므로 인간의 건강을 다루는 보건의료분야의 입문 단계에서 의학용어의 학습은 무엇보다도 중요하며 의료정보화 시대를 준비하는 핵심적인 과정으로써 보다 높은 의학에 대한 학습의 필요성이 절실한 실정이다.

이 책은 의학 및 간호보건계열 학생들이 전공분야를 학습하기 전에 기본적으로 알아두어야 할 의학용어의 일정한 특성을 파악하고 인체의 해부학·생리학·병리학의 전반적인 지식과 연계하여 의학용어를 쉽게 이해할 수 있도록 필요한 그림과 함께 연계하였다.

원고정리에 최선을 다하였으나 매듭을 짓고 나니 여전히 부족하고 미흡함이 눈에 거슬린다. 이러한 점들은 앞으로 여러 선배제현들의 지도편달을 받아 수정·보완해 나갈 것을 다짐 드리며, 각별한 성원과 배려를 바란다.

끝으로 이 책이 빛을 보기까지 격려해 주시고 많은 도움을 주신 여러분들께 깊이 감사를 드리며, 출판을 맡아 물심양면으로 애써 주신 고려의학 최병진 사장님과 편집부 직원들의 노고에 감사드립니다.

2008년 6월
저 자

CONTENTS

Chapter 1

BASIC MEDICAL TERMINOLOGY

I. Basic word structure

- Special vocabulary used by health care professionals for effective and accurate communication
- Based on Latin and Greek words
- Consistent and uniform throughout the world

1. Word root

- Fundamental unit of each medical word
    - Establishes basic meaning of word
    - Part to which prefixes and suffixes are added

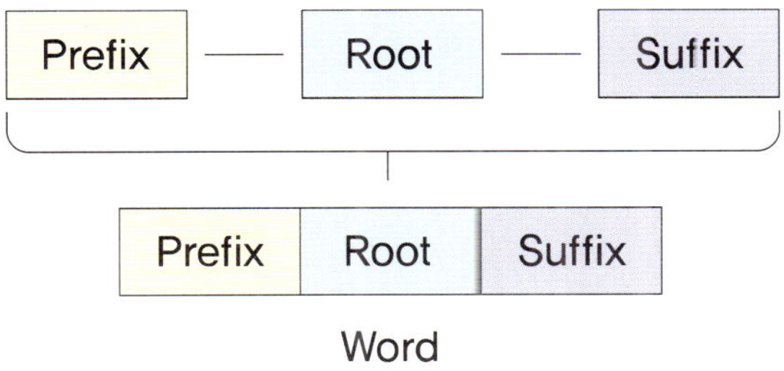

2. Prefix

- Short word part added before a root
    - Modifies the meaning of the root
    - Followed by a dash (*pre-*)

3. Suffix

- Short word part or parts added to the end of a word

- Modifies the meaning of the root
- Indicated by a dash before the suffix (- *itis*)

4. Combining vowel

- Roots shown with a combining vowel are called combining forms
    - Vowels added after a slash
    - Called roots
    - Neur/o
- Combining vowel omitted if suffix begins with a vowel
- Neur + it is = neuritis (inflammation of a nerve)

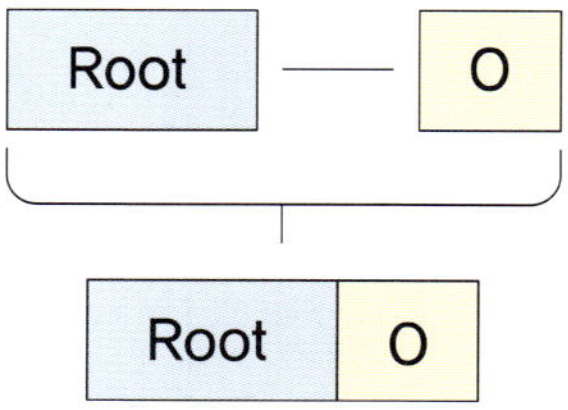

Combining form

5. Combining form

- The combination of a word root with the comvining vowel.

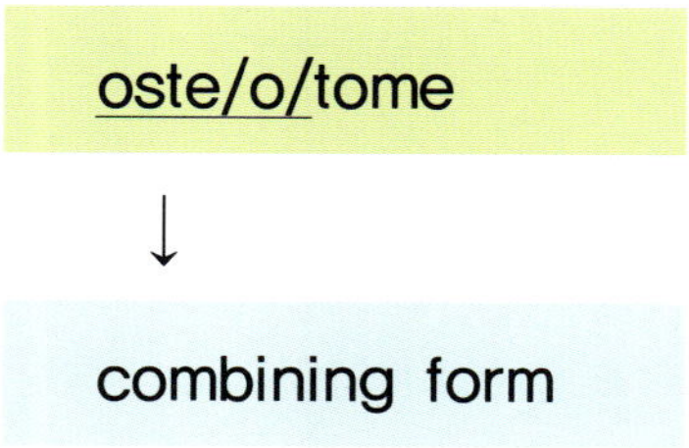

Ⅱ. Prefixes

■ Prefix = short word part added before a word root to modify the meaning

- *Uni-* (one) + *lateral* = *unilateral* (affecting or involving one side)
- *Contra-* (against) + *lateral* = *contralateral* (opposite side)

1. Prefixes involving site

Prefixes	Meaning	Term
ante, pre, pro(L)	before	antepituitary
cata, hypo(G)	under	catarrh
caud/o(L)	tail	caudad
cephal/o(G)	head	cephalad
dors/o(L)	back	dorsoflexion
en(em), endo(end)(G)	in	endoderm
ento, eso(G), intra(L)	in	intrasternal
epi, ep(G)	on	epidermis
exo, ecto(G), extra(L)	outside	ectoderm
latero(L)	side	lateroflexion
meso(G), mid(L)	middle	mesoderm
post, postero(L)	behind	postpituitary
supra(L)	above	suprasternal
ventr/i(ventr/o)(L)	abdomen	ventroflexion

2. Prefixes involving direction

Prefixes	Meaning	Term
a, de(L)	away	dementia
ab(L), apo(G)	away	abduction
ad(ac, af, ag)(L)	toward	adduction
ambi(ambo)(L), amphi(G)	both	ambidexter
antero, ante(L)	foreward	anterior
dextro(L)	right	dextrocardia
dia(G), per, trans(L)	through	diaphragm
dis(L), ap/o(G)	separation	disarticulation
ex(exo)(G, L)	outward	exostosis
in(im)(L)	into	infiltration
infer/o, infer/ior(L)	downward	inferior
inter(L)	between	intercostal
later/o(L)	to the side	lateroflexion
para(G)	beyond	paranasal
peri(G), circum(L)	around	circumduction
postero(L), retro(L)	backward	posterior
sinister(sinistr/o)(L)	left	sinistrocardia

3. Prefixes involving time and progress

Prefixes	Meaning	Term
acut/us(L)	sharp	acute
ante(L), pre(L), pro(G)	before	prognosis
brad/y(G)	slow	bradycardia
chron/o(G)	time	chronic
cycl/o(G)	recurring	cyclothymia
intra(L)	during	intraoperative
nyct/o(G), noct(L)	night	nyctalopia
post(L)	after	postoperative
tach/o(G)	speed	tachometer
tach/y(G)	rapid	tachycardia

4. Prefixes involving number

Prefixes	Meaning	Term
nulli(L), nullus(L)	none	nullipara
uni(L), mono, monus(G)	one	monocyte
primi, prima(L), prot/o(G)	first	primigravida
bi, amb(L), di(diplo)(G)	two	diplegia

tri(G, L)	three	tricepsmuscle
quadr/i(L), tetr/a(G)	four	tetralogy
quinque(L), pent/a(G)	five	pentalogy
hex/a(G)	six	hexadactylism
hept/a(G)	seven	heptadactylism
oct/a(oct/i)(G, L)	eight	octipara
nonus, noni(L), nona(G)	nine	nonus
deca(G)	ten	decagram
hect/o(G)	one hundred	hectometer
kil/o(G)	one thousand	kilometer
dec/i(L)	one tenth	decigram
cent/i(L)	one hundredth	centimeter
mill/i(L)	one thousandth	millimeter

5. Prefixes involving color

Prefixes	Meaning	Term
chlor/o(G)	green	chloroma
chrom/o(G), color(L)	color	chromosome
cyan/o(G)	blue	cyanosis
erythr/o(G), rubr/o(L)	red	erythrocyte
leuk/o(G), alba(albin/o)(L)	white	leukocyte
lute/o(L), flav/o(L)	yellow	luteinization
melan/o(G)	black	melanoderma
poli/o(G)	gray	poliomyelitis
purpur/o(L)	purple	purpura
xanth/o(G), cirrh/o(G)	orange	xanthoma

6. Prefixes involving structure

Prefixes	Meaning	Term
all/o(G)	reversal, another, other	allograft
ankyl/o(G)	bent, noose, loop	ankyloglossia
atel/o(G)	inperfect, incomplete	ateliosis
aut/o(L), idi/o(G)	self, own	autograft
cac, cac/o(G)	bad, ill	cachexia
cry/o(crym/o)(G)	cold	cryotherapy
crypt/o(G)	hidden, concealed, obscure	cryptorchism
dura(L), scirh/o, scler/o(G)	hard	duramater
dys(G)	difficult, bad, painful	dyspnea
eu(G)	well, good, easily	eupnea
febr/o(L), pyr/o, therm/o(G)	heat, fire	febrile
heter/o(G)	other, another	heterograft
hom/o(G), ipsi(L)	same	homograft
is/o(G)	equal	isograft
lept/o(G)	slender,thin	leptomeningioma
macro(G), magni(L)	large, big	macrocephalus
mal(L)	disease	malfunction
malac/o(G)	soft	malacia
mega(megal/o)(G)	large, big	megacolon
norm/o(L)	rule, usual, normal	normal
onc/o(G)	tumor, swelling, mass	oncology
orth/o(G)	stright, correct	orthopedics
pach/y(G)	thick	pachydermia
sten/o(G)	contracted, narrow	stenosis
terat/o(G)	malformation	teratoma
xen/o(G)	strange, foreign	xenograft
xer/o(G)	dry	xerostomia

7. Prefixes involving deny and confirm

Prefixes	Meaning	Term
a(an)(G)	without, not	anhidrosis
anti(G), contra(L)	against	antitoxin
con, co, com(L), syn(G)	together	congential
hemi(G)	one half	hemigastrectomy
hyper(G)	excessive, up	hyperglycemia
hypo(G)	deficient	hypoglycemia
in(im)(L)	not, lack	insomnia
olig/o(G)	few	oliguria
pan, pant/o(G)	all	pansinusitis
poly(G), multi(L)	many	polyuria
semi(L)	one half	semiplegia
sub(L)	almost	subluxation

Ⅲ. Suffixes

- Suffix = word ending that modifies a root
- May indicate a noun or adjective
- Often determines how word begins
  - *Myel / o* (bone marrow) + *-oid* = *meyloid* (like or pertaining to bone marrow)
  - *Myel / o* + *-oma* = *myeloma* (tumor of the bone marrow)

1. Suffixes involving condition

Suffixes	Meaning	Term
ia(G)	condition	leukemia
ism(G)	condition	hyperthyroidism
sis(G)	condition	hemolysis
asis(G)	condition	bronchiectasis
esis(G)	condition	pseudocyesis
iasis(G)	condition	lithiasis
osis(G)	condition	psychosis
sy(G)	disease, symptom	leprosy
us(L)	condition	anencephalus
y(G)	condition	anencephaly

2. Suffixes involving symptom (1)

Suffixes	Meaning	Term
algia(G), dynia(G)	pain	myalgia
carcinoma(G)	malignant tumor of epitherium cell	adenocarcinoma
cele(cel/o)(G)	herniation	cystocele
cyte(G)	cell	erythrocyte
emesis(G)	vomiting	hyperemesis
itis(G)	inflammation	neuritis
lithiasis(G)	stone	cholelithiasis
megaly(G)	enlargement	cardiomegaly
oma(G)	tumor, neoplasm, swelling	osteoma
pathy(G)	disease	encephalopathy
plasm, plasia(G)	formation	neoplasm
plegia(G)	paralysis, stroke	hemiplegia
plexy(G)	stroke	cataplexy
ptosis(G)	downward displacement	gastroptosis
rhage(rrhage)(G)	breaking, bursting forthh	hemorrhage
rhea(rrhea)(G)	flow, discharge	otorrhea
rhexis(rrhexis)(G)	rupture	enterorrhexis
sarcoma(G)	malignant tumor of connec-tive tissue and muscle	osteosarcoma
stasis, stasia(G)	stop	hemostasis
staxis(G)	hemorrhage	epistaxis

3. Suffixes involving symptom (2)

Suffixes	Meaning	Term
cyesis(G)	pregnancy	pseudocyesis
dipsia(G)	thirst	polydipsia
ectasia(ectasis)(G)	dilatation, expansion	bronchiectasia
emia(G)	blood	anemia
esthesia(G)	sense	anesthesia
logy(G)	study	histology
lysis(G)	destruction, separation	hysterolysis
malacia(G)	softening	osteomalacia
mnesia(G)	remember	amnesia
opia(G)	vision, see	diplopia
osis(G)	abnormal increase	leukocytosis
osmia(G)	small	anosmia
partum(L)	birth, labor	postpartum
penia(G)	abnormal reduction	leukopenia
pepsia(G)	digest	dyspepsia
phagia(G)	eat	polyphagia
philia(G)	abnormal fondness	pedophilia
phobia(G)	abnormal dread or fear	hydrophobia
phonia(G)	sound	aphonia
pnea(G)	breathe	hyperpnea
sclerosis(G)	hardening	arteriosclerosis
somnia(G)	sleep	insomnia
stenosis(G)	narrowing	bronchostenosis
trophy(G)	nourishment, development	atrophy

4. Suffixes involving surgical therapy

Suffixes	Meaning	Term
centesis(G), puncture(L)	perforation	thoracocentesis
clasis(clasia)(G)	surgical fracture	osteoclasis
clysis(G)	irrigation	rectoclysis
desis(G)	binding	arthrodesis
ectomy(G)	excision	gastroectomy
lapaxy(G), tripsy(G)	crushing, removal	litholapaxy
lysis(G)	separation	nephrolysis
pexy(G)	fixation	nephropexy
plasty(G)	surgical repair	rhinoplasty
rhaphy(rrhaphy)(G)	suture	blepharorrhaphy
stomy(G)	artificial opening	colostomy
tomy(G)	incision	laparotomy

5. Suffixes involving instrument and method

Suffixes	Meaning	Term
gram(G)	recorded	electroencephalogram
graph(G)	instrument for recording	electroencephalograph
graphy(G)	method of recording	electroencephalography
meter(G)	instrument for measuring	pelvimeter
metry(G)	method of measuring	pelvimetry
opsy(G)	vision	biopsy
scope(G)	instrument for examining	microscope
scopy(G)	method of examining	microscopy
tome(G)	instrument for cutting	osteotome
tomy(G)	method of cutting	laparotomy

Chapter 2

STRUCTURE OF THE BODY

I. Fundamental structure of the body

1. Cell

The cell is the fundamental unit of every living thing(animal or plant). Cells are every where in the human body-every tissue, every organ is made up of these individual units.

cell membrane : the structure surrounding and protecting the cell ; it determines what enters and leaves the cell.

nucleus : the structure that contains genetic material(chromosomes) and controls the activities of the cell.

cytoplasm : protoplasm that is outside the nucleus and within the cell membrane.

chromosomes : twenty-three pairs of rod-shaped structures in the nucleus ; each contains DNA.

2. Tissues

Tissues are groups of specialized cells.

epithelial tissue : the covering of internal and external surfaces of the body. Located all over the body as lining for internal organs, in exocrine and endocrine glands, and as the outer surface of skin covering the body.

muscle tissue : voluntary muscle is found in arms and legs and parts of the body where movement is voluntary, while involuntary muscle is found in the heart and digestive system, as well as other places where movement is not under conscious control.

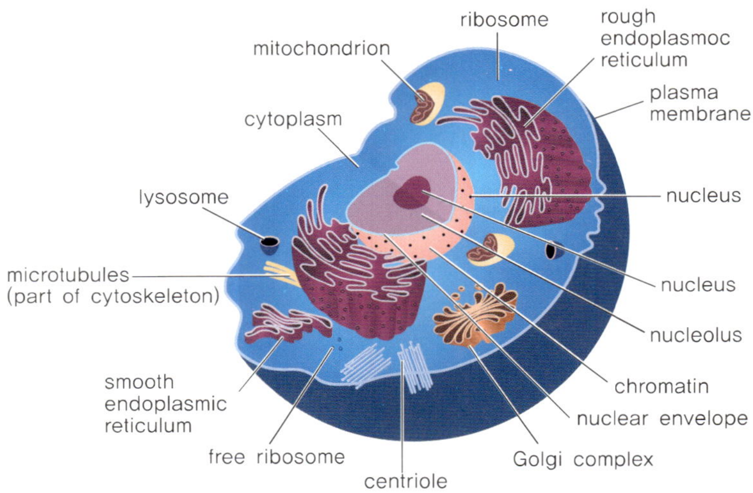

그림 2-1. The animal cell

connective tissue : the tissue which binds together and is the support of the various structures. This can be fat (also called adipose tissue), cartilage, bone, or blood.

nerve tissue : the substance of which the nerves and nerve centers are composed. Nerve tissue conducts impulses all over the body.

3. Organs

Organs are a somewhat independent part of the body that performs a special function. Organs are structures composed of several kinds of tissue. For example, an organ like the stomach is composed of muscle tissue, nerve tissue, and glandular epithelial tissue.

4. Systems

Systems are groups of organs working together in a common purpose.

Digestive system, Urinary system, Male reproductive system, Female reproductive system, Nervous system, Psychoneural system, Cardiovascular system, Blood and Lymphatic system, Respiratory system, Musculoskeletal system, Endocrine system, Integumentary system, Auditory system, Visual system.

Ⅱ. Body cavities

A body cavity is a space within the body which contains internal organs(viscera).

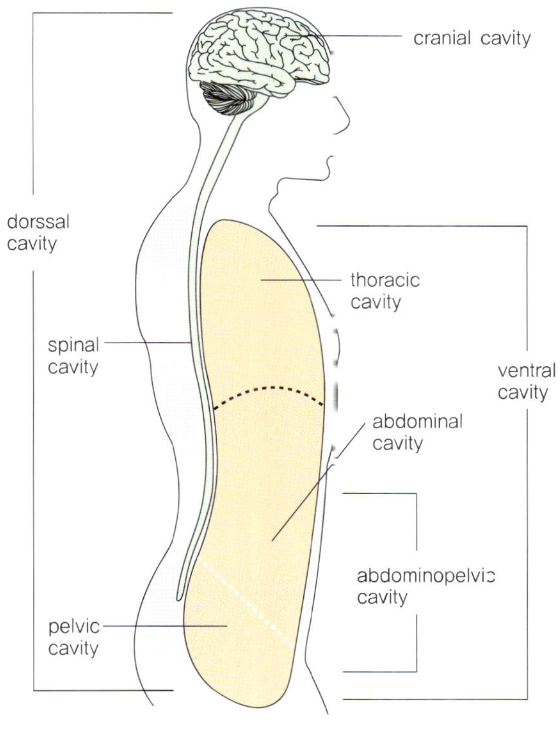

그림 2-2. Body cavities

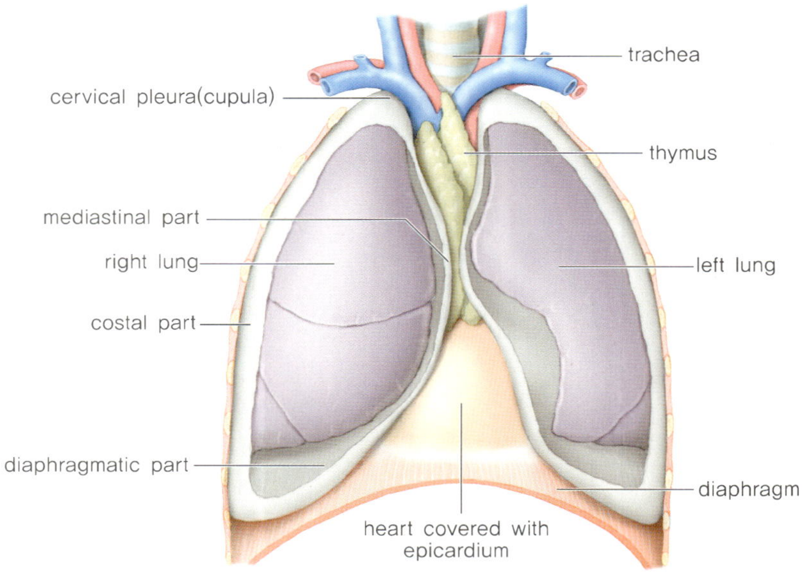

그림 2-3. Divisions of the thoracic cavity

1. Cranial cavity

The space enclosed by the bones of the cranium.

2. Thoracic cavity

The ventral body cavity situated between the neck and the respiratory diaphragm.

(1) Pleural cavity

The areas surrounding the lungs.

(2) Mediastinum

The area between the lungs.

3. Abdominal cavity

The cavity of the body located between the diaphragm and the pelvis.

4. Pelvic cavity

The space within the walls of the pelvis.

5. Spinal cavity

Nerves of spinal cord.

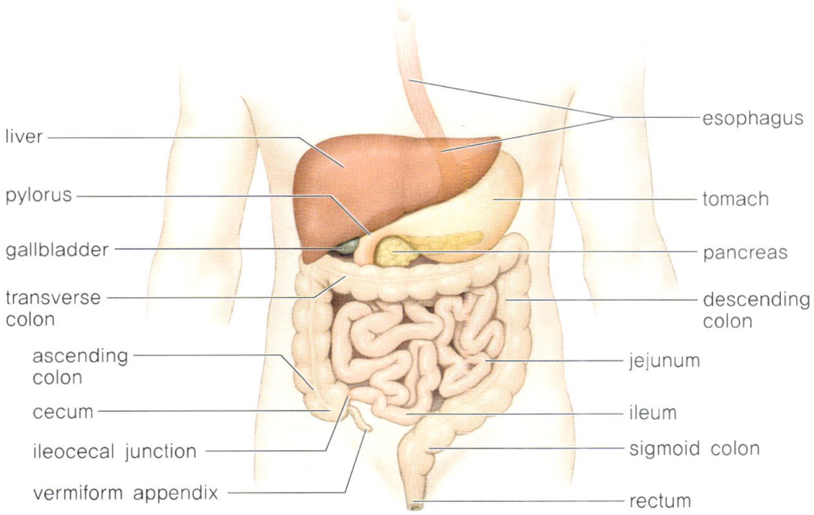

그림 2-4. Organs of the peritoneum and abdominal cavity

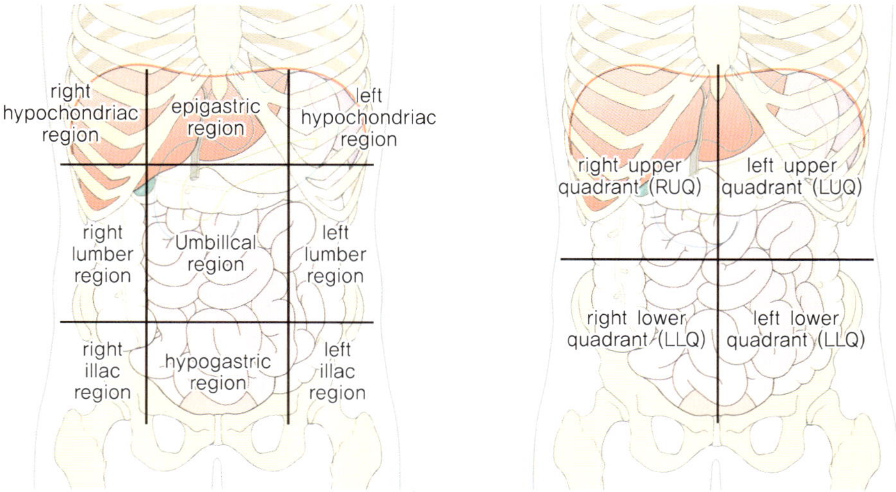

그림 2-5. Anatomical divisions of the abdomen

Ⅲ. Divisions of the abdomen and back

1. Anatomical divisions of the abdomen

(1) Hypochondriac regions

The upper lateral region of the abdomen, on either side of the epigastric region.

(2) Epigastric region

The upper middle region of the abdomen.

(3) Lumbar region

The middle lateral region of the abdomen.

(4) Umbilical region

The region of umbilicus.

(5) Inguinal(iliac) regions

The lower lateral region of the abdomen.

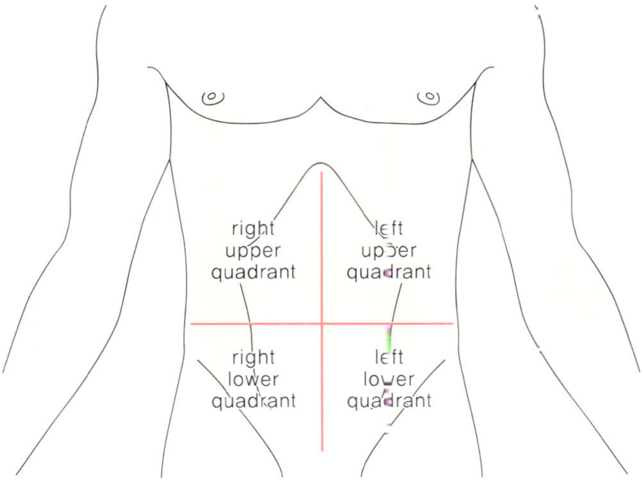

그림 2-6. Clinical divisions of the abdomen

(6) Hypogastric region

The lower middle region, below the umbilical region.

2. Clinical divisions of the abdomen

(1) Right upper quadrant(RUQ)

Liver, gallbladder, right kidney, etc.

(2) Left upper quadrant(LUQ)

Stomach, pancreas, spleen, left kidney, etc.

(3) Right lower quadrant(RLQ)

Cecum, vermiform appendix, right ureter, ascending colon, right ovary and uterine tube, etc.

(4) Left lower quadrant(LLQ)

Left ureter, descending colon, sigmoid colon, left ovary and uterine tube, etc.

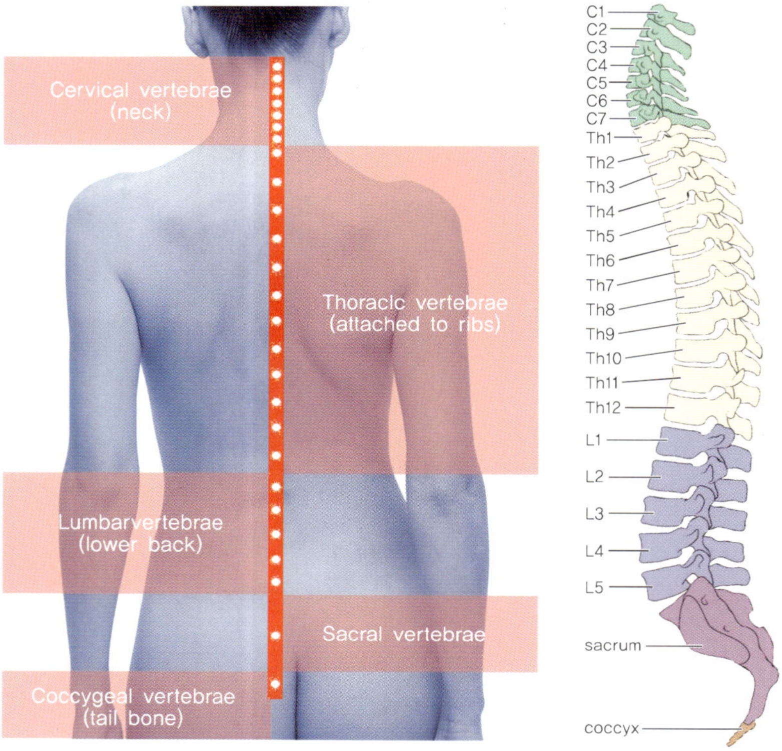

그림 2-7. Anatomical divisions of the back (spinal column)

3. Anatomical divisions of the back(spinal column)

(1) Cervical regions

Neck region(C1 - C7).

(2) Thoracic regions

Chest region(T1 - T12, D1 - D12 : dorsal).

(3) Lumbar regions

Loin region(L1 - L5).

(4) Sacral regions

Sacrum region(S1 - S5).

(5) Coccygeal regions

Coccyx region(tail bone).

IV. Anatomic positions and body regions

1. Anatomic positions

There are numerous terms to describe anatomic positions. Some of the more frequently used are listed, below;

erect : standing position.

knee-chest : kneeling with chest resting on table(genupectoral position).

lateral recumbent : lying on left side with right thigh and knee drawn up (Sim's position).

prone : lying face down, ventral recumbent.

supine : lying flat on back, dorsal recumbent.

2. Body regions

(1) Thorax and abdomen

axillary : armpit (axilla) and its borders.

clavicular : region on either side of the breastbone (sternum), extending the length of the clavicles.

epigastric : area within the costal arch (arch of the rib cage), which is in the median part of the surface of the abdomen.

hypochondriac : areas, right and left, of the epigastric region.

hypogastric : region in the lower abdomen between the inguinal regions and lying between and below the iliac spines.

infraclavicular : area below the clavicles.

inguinal : or iliac regions, triangular in shape, on either side of the hypogastric region.

lateral abdominal : regions lying on either side of the umbilical region.

mammary : region on either side of the chest between the third and sixth ribs, extending below the lower margins of the pectoralis major muscles on either side; the breasts are in this region.

pubic : region in the central portion of the hypogastric region above the pubis.

sternal : area over the front of the sternum.

subinguinal : regions just below the inguinal region.

supraclavicular : area above the clavicles.

umbilical : medical abdominal region, above the hypogastric.

(2) Posterior trunk

coxal : areas just below the lumbar regions in the back and lateral abdominal regions on either side: they are bordered by the gluteal regions (area over the buttocks)

infrascapular : area on either side, extention down to the last rib.

interscapular : part of the medial region of the back, between the scapulae and on either side of the vertebral column.

lumbar : region immediately below the infrascapular region and extention down to the crest of the ilium.

medial region of back : central zone of the back, extention from the region of the neck as far down as the base of sacrum.

nuchal : region of back of neck that begins just below the occipital region of the head and extends down to the spine of the seventh cervical vertebra.

sacral : area over the sacrum at the base of the median region.

suprascapular : areas on either side above the scapular region and extending to the curve of the neck.

(3) Head

auricular : region around the ears.

buccal : region of the cheeks.

infraorbital : region immediately below the eyes.

mental : region of the chin.

occipital : region covering the occipital bone.

orbital : region around the eyes.

submaxillary : region on either side of the submental region below the ramus of the mandible.

submental : region below the chin.

supraorbital : region above the eyebrows.

V. Planes and lines of the body

The anatomic position of the body is erect, with the arms at the sides and the palms turned forward, Many of the terms established to describe location or position of parts are based on this body position

A plane is an imaginary flat surface.

- Frontal plane
  - Coronal plane
  - Divides body into anterior, posterior parts
- Sagittal plane
  - Divides body into right, left portions
  - If plane cuts midline, called midsagittal or medial plane
- Transverse plane
  - Divides body into superior, inferior parts

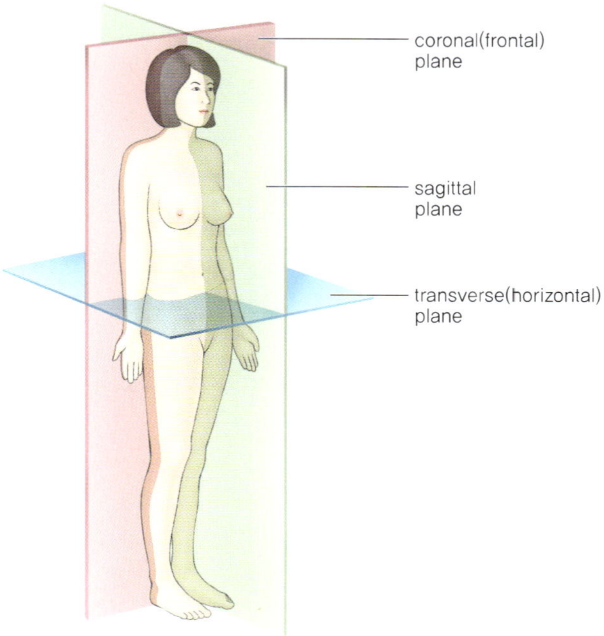

그림 2-8. Planes of the body(The figure is standing in the anatomical position)

Infraorbitomeatal line : the line connecting between the infraorbital margin and external acoustic meatus.

Interpupillary line : the line connecting between the pupils.

Orbitomeatal line : the line connecting between the orbit and external acoustic meatus.

Acanthiomeatal line : the line connecting between the acanthion and external acoustic meatus.

Glabellomeatal line : the line connecting between the glabella and external acoustic meatus.

Glabelloalveolar line : the line connecting between the glabella and alveolus.

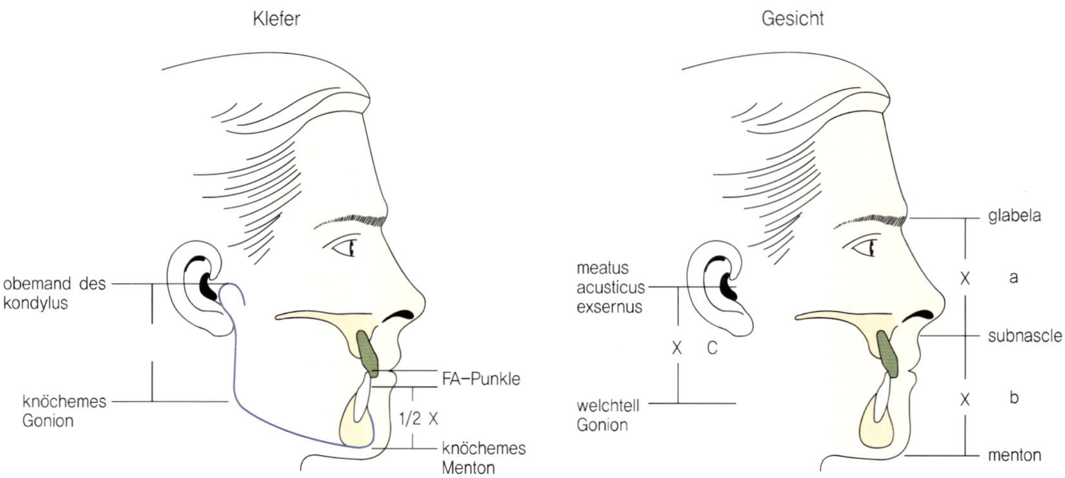

그림 2-9. Basic localization points and lines

VI. Terms of the direction and movement

1. Type of direction

afferent : conducting toward a structure.

anterior or ventral : front of the body (not synonymous in lower limb).

central : toward the center.

deep : away from the surface.

distal or peripheral : away from the beginning of a structure; away from the center.

efferent : conducting away from a structure.

inferior or caudal : away from the head, situated below another structure.

intermediate : between median and lateral.

lateral : toward the side.

medial : toward the median plane.

median : in the middle of a structure.

posterior or dorsal : back of the body (not synonymous in lower limb).

proximal : toward the beginning of a structure.

superficial : near the surface.

superior or cephalic : toward head end of body.

2. Type of movement

flexion : bending at a joint, as the forearm or elbow.

extension : straightening, or unbending, of a joint; this movement is the opposite of flexion.

abduction : movement that draws a body part away from the midline of the body, such as the extension of the arms straight out from the shoulders.

adduction : movement that draws the body part toward the midline of the body, such as returning extended arms to side.

rotation : movement that turns a body part on its own axis ; for example, the turning of the head.

pronation : turning down or downward ; for example, turning the palm of the hand downward.

supination : turning upward ; for example, turning the palm upward.

eversion : turn outward.

inversion : turning inward.

VII. Unfamiliar root words for body parts and organs

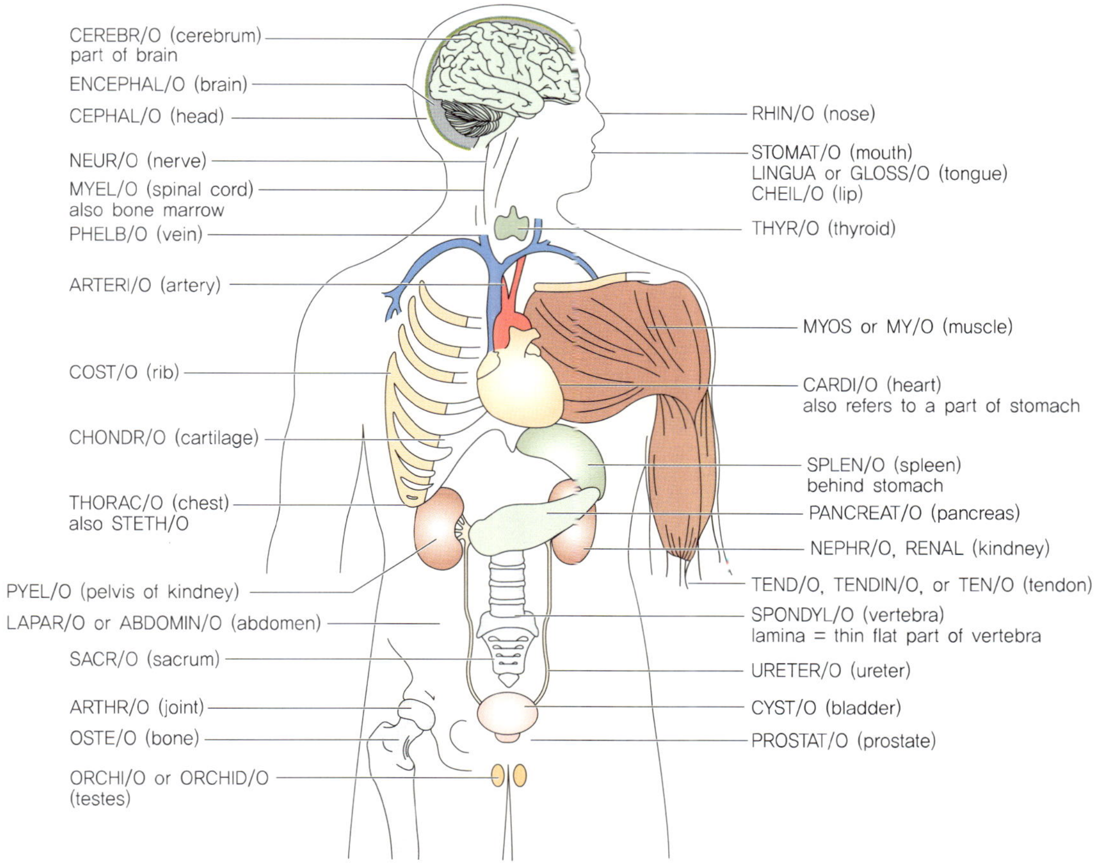

그림 2-10. Andro(man). Anterior view, partial skeleton shown; abdominal viscera not show. Showing male reproductive organs, urinary tract, heart, spleen, pancreas, hip joint, and some shoulder muscles.

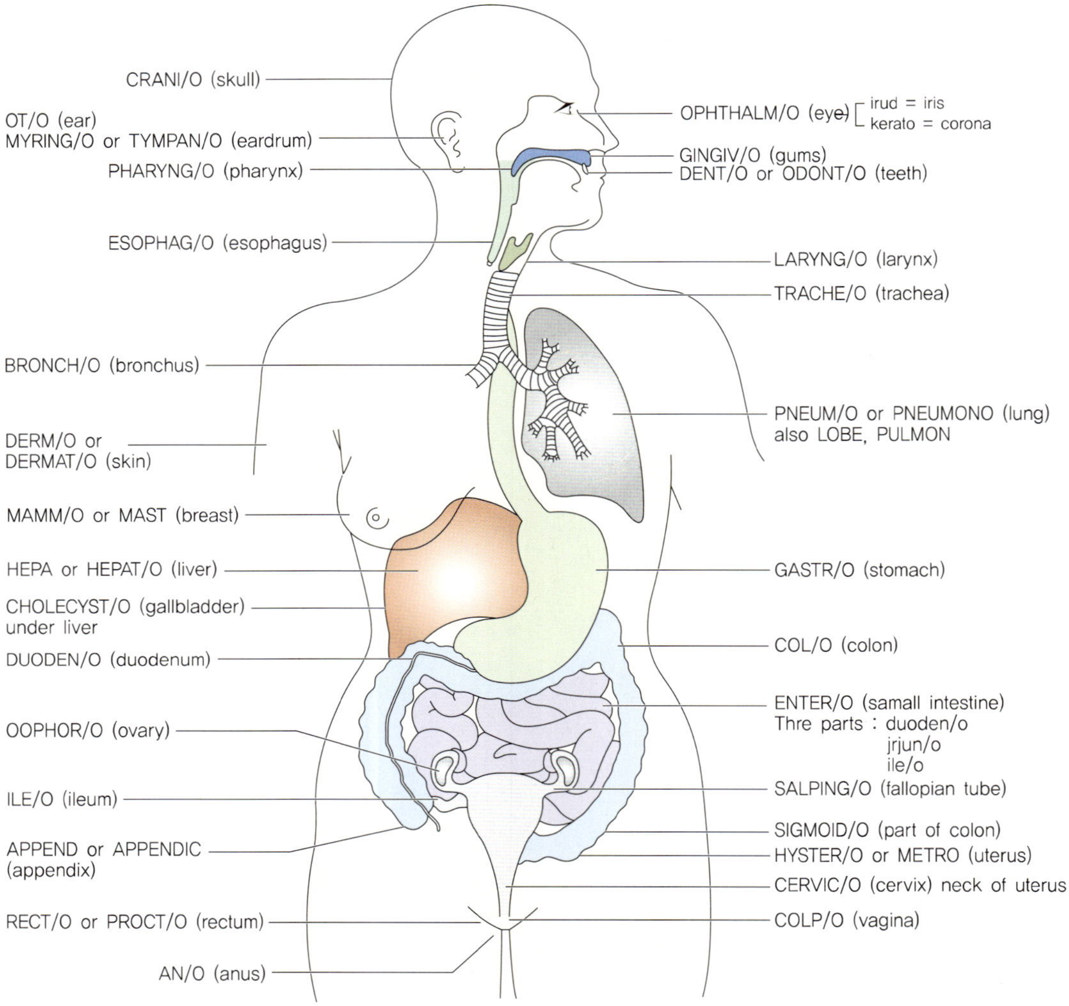

그림 2-11. Gyne(woman). Anterior view, no body structure shown. Showing intestinal tract, female reproductive organs.

Chapter

3

DIGESTIVE SYSTEM

Gastrointestinal system functions : ingestion, digestion, and absorption of food or nutritive elements. The gastrointestinal(GI) system is also called the digestive system.

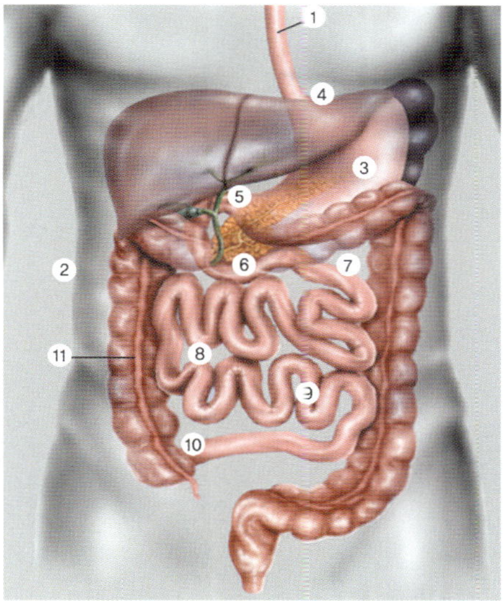

① The esophagus is a long muscular tube, which moves food from the mouth to the stomach.
② The abdomen contains all of the digestive organs.
③ The stomach, situated at the top of the abdomen, normally holds just over 3 pints (about 1500 ml) of food from a single meal. Here the food is mixedwith an acid that is produced to assist in digestion. In the stomach, acid and other digestive juices are added to the ingested food to facilitate breakdown of complex proteins, fats and carbohydrates into small, more absorbable units.
④ A valve at the entrance to the stomach from the esophagus allows the food to enter while keeping the acid-laden food from "refluxing" back into the esophagus, causing damage and pain.
⑤ The pylorus is a small round muscle located at the outlet of the stomach and the entrance to the duodenum (the first section of the small intestine). It closes the stomach outlet while food is being digested into a smaller, more easily absorbed form. When food is properly digested, the pylorus opens and allows the contents of the stomach into the duodenum.
⑥ The small intestine is about 15 to 20 feet long (4.5 to 6 meters) and is where the majority of the absorption of the nutrients from food takes place. The small intestine is made up of three sections: the duodenum, the jejunum and the ileum.
⑦ The duodenum is the first section of the small intestine and is where the food is mixed with bile produced by the liver and with other juices from the pancreas. This is where much of the iron and calcium is absorbed.
⑧ The jejunum is the middle part of the small intestine extending from the duodenum to the ileum: it is responsible for digestion.
⑨ The last segment of the intestine, the ileum, is where the absorption of fat-soluble vitamins A, D, E and K and other nutrients are absorbed.
⑩ Another valve separates the small and large intestines to keep bacteria-laden colon contents from coming back into the small intestine.
⑪ In the large intestines, excess fluids are absorbed and a firm stool is formed. The colon may absorb protein, when necessary.

그림 3-1. Gastrointestinal organs showing, some pathologic conditions: peptic ulcer, diverticulosis, polyp, and hemorrhoid.

organs through which food passes : alimentary canal.

mouth : oral cavity.

pharynx : it serve as a common passage way for air from the nasal cavity to the larynx as well as for food going from the mouse to the esophagus.

esophagus : muscular tube extending from the pharynx to the stomach.

stomach : cardiac sphincter at entrance ; pyloric sphincter at exit(greater and lesser curvatures-large and small outer walls of stomach). Do not confuse "stomach" and "abdomen."

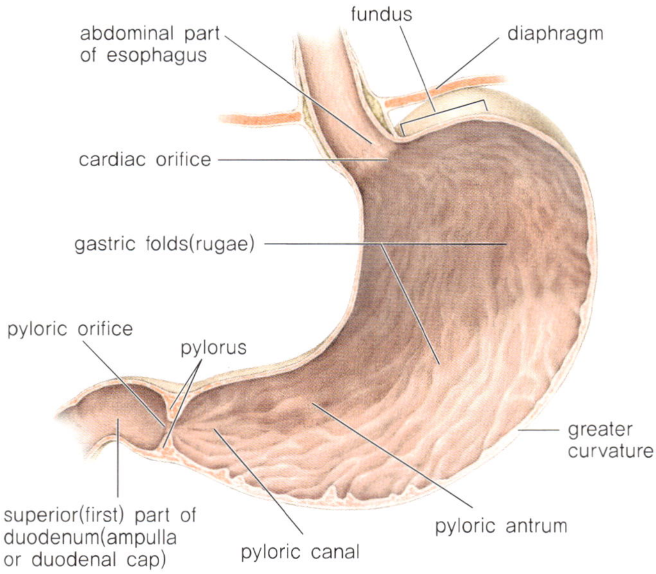

그림 3-2. The stomach

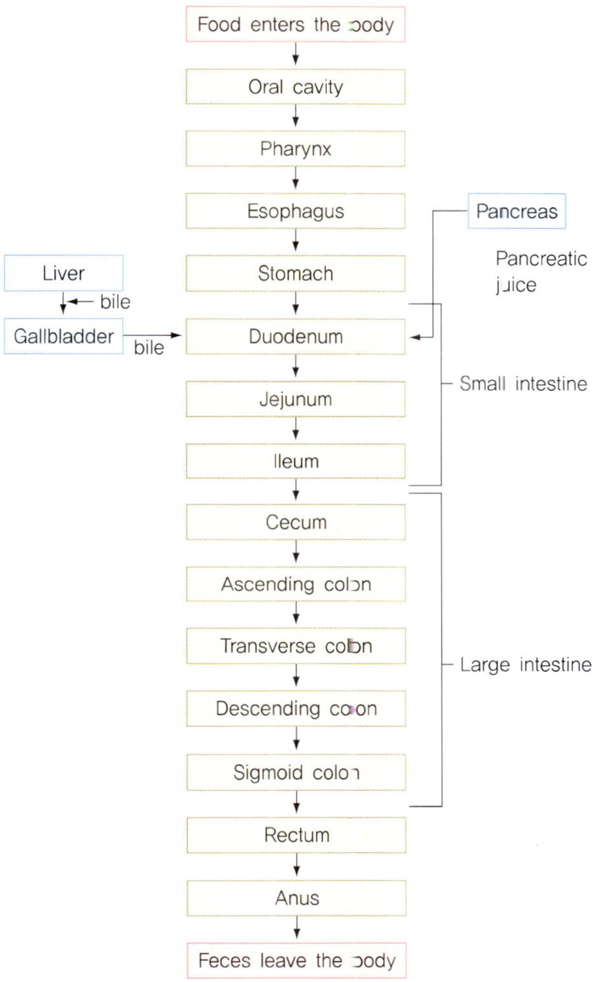

그림 3-3. Pathway of food through the digestive tract

duodenum, jejunum, ileum : small intestine, three parts ; ileocecal valve prevents contents of large bowel from reentering small intestine.

cecum : appendix attached ; first part of large intestine.

ascending colon : large intestine. Hepatic flexure where ascending colon turns into.

transverse colon : large intestine. Splenic flexure where transverse colon turns into.

descending colon : large intestine.

sigmoid colon : large intestine.

rectum : large intestine.

anus : anal sphincter(sphincter muscle is circular, like a purse string).

Digestion

mechanical process : food is broken up, mixed with digestive juices. It is moved along by peristalsis(rhythmic contraction of the intestines).

chemical process : food reacts with enzymes. Large molecules are broken down so they can pass through the mucous membrane into the blood and from there to the cells.

absorption : takes place in the small intestines. Villi, which are tiny projections lining intestines, provide large surface area through which nutrients can be absorbed.

elimination : of solid wastes in the form of feces. Also called fecal matter, stool, and bowel movement.

metabolism : the sum of all physical and chemical changes that take place within the body and all energy and transformations that occur within cells; change of food to mechanical energy or heat.

nutrients : food ; proteins, fats, carbohydrates, plus vitamins and essential minerals. Proteins and carbohydrates(CHO) contain 4 calories per gram; fats contain 9 calories per gram. Protein is essential for growth and repair of tissue. Fats and carbohydrates provide heat and energy.

Essential vitamins : A, B_1(thiamine), B_2(riboflavin), niacin, B_6 (pyridoxine), B_{12}(cyanocobalamin), C(ascorbic acid), D folic acid, and K.

Essential minerals : calcium, iron, iodine, zinc, copper, magnesium, potassium, phosphorus, sodium.

Areas of abdomen

quadrants : four divisions : RUQ, RLQ, LUQ and LLQ.

divisions : nine sections.

1. Right and left hypochondria.
2. Right and left lumbar.
3. Right and left inguinal or iliac.
4. Epigastric.
5. Umbilical.
6. Suprapubic or hypogastric.

Accessory organs

teeth : incisors(central and lateral) ; cuspids or canines ; bicuspids or premolars ; and molars(first and second) ; third are "wisdom" teeth.

tongue : muscular organ, covered with mucous membrane ; taste buds are present on surfaces of papillae.

salivary glands : three pairs ; parotid, sublingual and submandibular.

pancreas : behind stomach ; excretes pancreatic juice to duodenum(papilla of Vater) ; also secretes the hormone insulin into blood(function of endocrine system).

liver : largest gland(RUQ) ; responsible for hundreds of chemical reactions.

1. Stores fats and sugars ; makes proteins(albumin, globbulins, cholesterol).
2. Secretes bile(essential for digestion of fats).

Digestive System

3. Regulates blood sugar.
4. Removes wastes from blood ; detoxifies substances.

gallbladder : behind liver ; stores and concentrates bile. Hepatic ducts drain bile from liver ; cystic duct by which bile enters and leaves gallbladder ; common bile duct, union of these two, into duodenum(by way of ampulla of Vater at sphincter of Oddi). The common bile duct and pancreatic duct meet to enter the duodenum.

I. Oral cavity

1. Word root

alveol/o	alveolar
bucc/o	cheek
cheil/o, labi/o	lip
dent/o, odont/o	tooth
gingiv/o	gum
gloss/o, lingu/o	tongue
mandibl/o	lower jaw
or/o, stomat/o	mouth
palat/o	palate
parotid/o	beside the ear
pharyng/o	throat
ptyal/o, sial/o	saliva
sialaden/o	salivaly gland
tonsill/o	tonsil
uvul/o, staphyl/o	uvula

2. Anatomical terms

alveolus	gingiva
buccal cavity	labium
cement	palate
cervix dentis	pulp
corona dentis	radix dentis
dentin	tongue, linguae
enamel	uvula
fauces	velum palatinum
frenulum linguae	

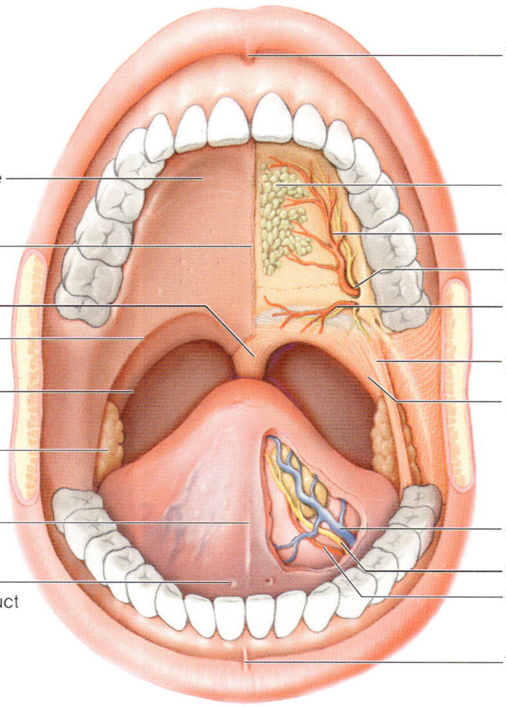

그림 3-4. Oral cavity

Bartholin's duct	saliva
glandulae buccales	Stensen's duct
glandulae labiales	sublingual gland
glandulae palatinae	submandibular gland
lingual gland	Wharton's duct
parotid gland	

3. Medical terms

Abbe-Estlander operation : the transfer of a full thickness flap from one lip to fill a defect in the other lip.

ankyloglossia : tongue tie.

aphtha : small ulcers, especially the whitish or reddish spots in the mouth characteristic of aphthous stomatitis.

aptyalism : deficiency or absence of the saliva.

avulsion : a tearing away of a part of structure.

candidasis : infection by fungi of the genus Candida, generally candida albicans, most commonly involving the skin, oral mucosa (thrush), respiratory tract, and vagina; rarely there is systemic infection or endocarditis. Called also moniliasis.

canker : an ulceration, especially of the lip or oral mucosa.

caries : the molecular decay or death of a bone, in which it becomes softened, discolored, and porous.

cheilitis : inflammation of the lips.

cheiloplasty : surgical repair of a lip defect.

cheilorrhaphy : the operation of suturing the lip.

cheilostomatoplasty : surgical restoration of the lips and mouth.

cleft palate : a fissure or elongated opening, especially one occurring in the embryo or derived from a failure of the roof of the mouth to fuse during embryonic development.

edentia : absence of the teeth.

frenotomy : incision of a frenulum, as of the frenulum linguae in treatment of tongue-tie.

gingivitis : a general term for inflammation of the gums, of which bleeding is one of the primary symptoms. Other symptoms include swelling, redness, pain and difficulty in chewing.

glossectomy : excision of all or a portion of the tongue.

glossitis : inflammation of the tongue.

glossocele : swelling and protrusion of the tongue.

glossodynia : pain in the tongue.

glossoplasty : plastic operation on the tongue.

glossorrhaphy : suture of the tongue.

halitosis : offensive odor of the breath.

harelip : a congenital cleft or defect in the upper lip, usually due to failure of the median nasal and maxillary processes to unite.

leukoplakia : a disease marked by the development on the mucous membranes of the cheeks, gums, or tongue of white thickened patches which sometimes show a tendency to fissure and have a pronounced tendency to become malignant.

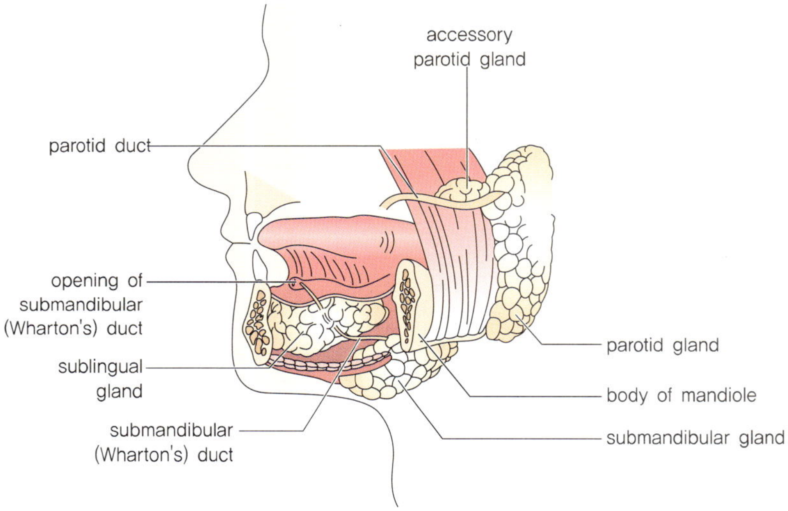

그림 3-5. Salivary glands

Ludwigs angina : diffuse purulent inflammation around the submaxillary gland, beneath the jaw, and about the floor of the mouth, usually due to streptococcal infection.

moniliasis : a superficial infection of the moist cutaneous areas of the body.

mumps : a communicable paramyxovirus disease that attacks one or both of parotid gland, the largest of the three pairs of salivary gland; called also epidemic parotitis.

odontalgia, dentalgia : pain in a tooth.

odontectomy : excision of an erupted or impacted tooth.

odontoma : any tumor of odontogenic origin.

palatoplasty : plastic reconstruction of the palate.

palatorrhaphy : surgical correction of a cleft palate.

parotidectomy : excision of a parotid gland.

parotitis, paritiditis : inflammation of the parotid gland.

pharyngalgia : pain in the pharynx.

pharyngectomy : surgical removal of a part of the pharynx.

pharyngitis : acute inflammation of the pharynx.

ptyalectasis : dilatation of a salivary duct.

ptyalism : excessive secretion of saliva.

restorative : promoting a return to health or to consciousness.

sialoadenitis : inflammation of a salivary gland.

sialoadenotomy, sialadenotomy : incision and drainage of a salivary gland.

sialography : demonstration of the salivary ducts by means of the injection of contrast medium.

sialolithiasis : the formation of salivary calculi.

sialolithotomy : incision of a salivary calculi.

sore : a popular term for any lesion of the skin or mucous membrane.

stomalgia, stomatodynia : pain in the mouth.

stomatitis : inflammation of the mucosa of the mouth.

stomatorrhagia : hemorrhage from the mouth.

stomatoplasty : plastic surgery of, or operative repair of, defects of the mouth or of the osteum uteri.

thrush : infection of the oral mucous membrane by a fungus(candida albicans).

tonsillectomy : surgical removal of a tonsil or tonsils.

tonsillitis : acute inflammation of the palatine tonsils.

tonsillolith : calculus in a tonsil.

uvulitis : inflammation of the uvula.

Vincent's angina : gingivostomatitis caused by extension to the oral mucosa of necrotizing ulcerative gingivitis(trench mouth), char acterized by ulceration, pseudomembrane, and odor, with lesions involving the palate or pharynx as well as the oral mucosa.

xerostomia : dryness of the mouth from lack of the normal secretion.

Ⅱ. Esophagus and stomach

1. Word root

cardi/o	cardia
esophag/o	esophagus
gastr/o	stomach
muc/o	mucus
pylor/o	pylorus
-ectasis	dilatation
-emesis	vomiting
-pepsia	digestion
-phagia	swallow
-prandial	meal
-stenosis	narrowing
-tresis	perforation

2. Anatomical terms

angular incisure	omentum
cardia	pharynx
diaphragm	pyloric antrum
esophagus	pylorus
fundus	stomach
greater curvature	rugae
lesser curvature	

3. Medical terms

achalasia : failure to relax of the smooth muscle fibers of the gastrointestinal tract at any junction of one part with another; especially failure of the lower esophagus to relax with swallowing. dut to degeneration of ganglion cells in the wall of the organ.

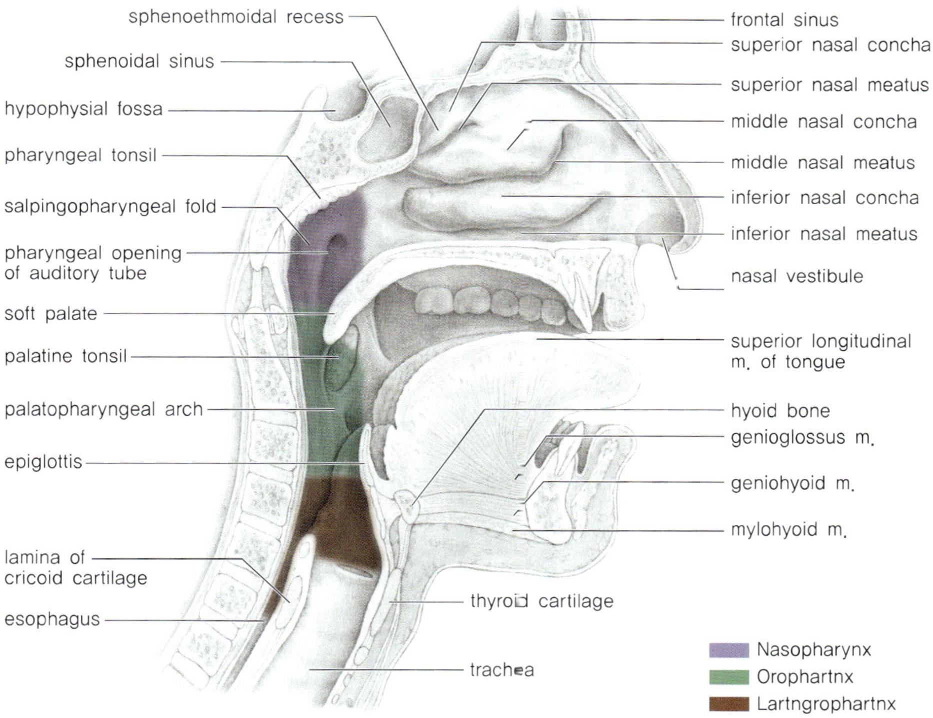

그림 3-6. Pharynx

achlorhydria : absence of hydrochloric acid from gastric juice ; associated with pernicious anemia, stomach cancer, and pellagra.

anorexia : lack or loss of appetite for food.

antrectomy : excision of an antrum.

aphagia : loss of the power of swallowing.

bulimia : abnormal increase in the sensation of hunger.

Crohn's disease : a chronic granulomatous inflammatory disease of unknown etiology.

diverticulectomy : excision of a diverticulum.

diverticulitis : inflammation of a diverticulum, especially inflammation involving diverticula of the colon.

diverticulosis : the presence of diverticula in the absence of inflammation.

dumping syndrome : nausea, weakness, sweating, palpitation, syncope, often a sensation of warmth, and sometimes diarrhea, occurring after ingestion of food in patients who have had partial gastrectomy.

dyspepsia : indigestion, cacochymia, impairment of the power or function of digestion.

dysphagia : difficulty in swallowing.

epigastric pain : the pain in the upper middle region of the abdomen.

eructation : the oral ejection of gas or air from the stomach; belching.

esophageal perforation : a hole made through the inner surface of the esophagus.

esophagectomy : excision of a portion of the esophagus.

esophagitis : inflammation of the esophagus.

esophagoenterostomy : anastomosis between the esophagus and small intestine.

esophagogastrostomy : anastomosis of the esophagus to the stomach.

esophagoscopy : direct visual examination of the esophagus with an esophagoscope.

fluroscope : an instrument for visual observation of the form and motion of the deep structures of the body by means of X-ray. Examination by this method is called fluroscopy.

gastrectomy : excision of the stomach(total gastrectomy) or a portion of it(partial or subtotal gastrectomy).

gastric ulcer : an ulceration of the mucous membrane of the stomach.

gastritis : inflammation of the lining of the stomach.

gastrointestinal series : an examination of the upper gastrointestinal tract using barium as the contrast medium for a series of X-ray films, called also a barium meal.

gastrojejunostomy : anastomosis between the stomach and jejunum.

gastrolavage : irrigation of the stomach.

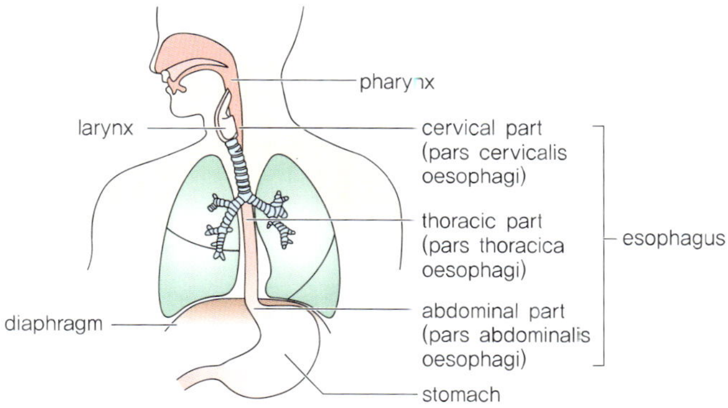

그림 3-7. Esophagus

gastropexy : surgical fixation of the stomach.

gastroptosis : downward displacement of the stomach.

gastroscopy : inspection of the interior of the stomach with a gastro scope.

gastrostomy : surgical creation of an artificial opening into the stomach.

gavage : forced feeding, especially through a tube passed into the stomach ; called also tube feeding.

hematemesis : the vomiting of blood.

hernia : the abnormal protrusion of part of an organ or tissue through the structures normally containing it.

hyperacidity, hyperchylia : an excessive degree of acidity.

hypertrophy of Brunner's gland : hypertrophy of the tubuloalveolar glands in the submucous layer of the duodenum.

hypochlorhydria : deficiency of hydrochloric acid in the gastric juice.

lavage : irrigation or washing out of an organ or cavity, as of the stomach or intestine.

Loreta's operation : gastrotomy with distal dilatation of the pylorus.

nausea : an unpleasant sensation vaguely referred to the epigastrium and abdomen, with a tendency to vomit.

peptic ulcer : an ulceration of the mucous membrane of the esophagus, stomach, or jejunum.

pyloric stenosis : obstruction of the pyloric orifice of the stomach, it may be congenital as in hypertrophic pyloric stenosis, or acquired, due to peptic ulceration or prepyloric carcinoma.

pylorodiosis : the operation of dilating a stricture of the pylorus with the finger.

pyloroplasty : a plastic operation to relieve pyloric obstruction.

pyrosis : heartburn; a burning sensation in the esophagus and stomach, with sour eructation.

ulcer : a local defect, or excavation of the surface of an organ or tissue, produced by sloughing of necrotic inflammatory tissue. As commonly used, the term often refers to a peptic ulcer of the inner wall, of lining, of the stomach(gastric ulcer) or of the duodenum(duodenal ulcer).

regurgitation : a backward flowing, as the casting up of undigested food, or the backflow of blood through a defective heart valve.

vagotomy : interruption of the impulses carried by the vagus nerve or nerves ; so called because it was first performed by surgical methods. The surgical procedure is done as part of the treatment of gastric or duodenal ulcer and often is performed in combination with gastroenterostomy or partial gastrectomy.

vomiting : forcible ejection of contents of stomach through the mouth.

Whipple's operation : radical pancreaticoduodenectomy.

Zollinger-Ellison syndrome : a triad comprising intractable, sometimes fulminating, atypical peptic ulcers; extreme gastric hyperacidity; and nonbeta-cell, gastric-secreting islet cell tumors(gastrinomas) of the pancreas which might be single or multiple, small or large, benign or malignant.

Ⅲ. Small and large intestine

1. Word root

aer/o	air
an/o	anus
append/o, appendic/o	appendix
cec/o	cecum
celi/o, lapar/o	abdomen
col/o, colon/o	colon
copr/o	feces, stool
diverticul/o	diverticulum
duoden/o	duodenum
enter/o	small intestine
epipl/o	omentum
ile/o	ileum
jejun/o	jejunum
omphal/o	umbilicus
proct/o	anus and rectum
rect/o	rectum
sigmoid/o	sigmoid colon

2. Anatomical terms

anus	jejunum
appendix	large intestine
cecum	McBurney's point
colon	rectum
diverticulum	small intestine
duodenum	umbilicus
ileum	

3. Medical terms

anal fissure : tear or ulcer at the margin of the anus.

anal fistula : opening in the anal canal and the perianal skin.

anal stenosis : stricture of the anus.

anoplasty : a plastic or restorative operation on the anus.

appendectomy : excision of the vermiform appendix.

appendicitis : inflammation of the vermiform appendix.

borborygmus : a rumbling noise caused by propulsion of gas through the intestines.

cecectomy : excision of the cecum.

colectomy : excision of the colon or of a portion of it.

colic : acute paroxysmal abdominal pain.

colitis : inflammation of the colon.

colocolostomy : surgical formation of an anastomosis between two portions of the colon.

colopexy : surgical fixation or suspension of the colon.

coloproctectomy : surgical removal of the colon and rectum.

colostomy : an artificial opening(stoma) created in the large intestine and brought to the surface of the abdomen for the purpose of evacuating the bowels; also the opening(stoma) so created.

constipation : ordinarily a condition in which the waste matter in the bowels is too hard to pass easily, or in which bowel movements are infrequent that discomfort or uncomfortable symptoms result.

dehydration : excessive loss of body water.

diarrhea : rapid movement of fecal matter through the intestine resulting in poor absorption of water, nutritive elements, and electrolyte and producing abnormally frequent evacuation of watery stools.

diverticulitis : inflammation of a diverticulum.

Duhamel operation : the treatment of Hirschsprung's disease.

duodenectomy : excision of the duodenum.

duodenitis : inflammation of the duodenum.

duodenojejunostomy : surgical communication between the duodenum and the jejunum.

dysentery : any of a number of disorders marked by inflammation of the intestine, especially of the colon, with abdominal pain, tenesmus, and frequent stools often containing blood and mucus.

enterectomy : excision of a portion of the intestine.

enteritis : inflammation of the small intestine.

enteroclysis : the injection of a nutrient or liquid into the bowel.

enterocolostomy : surgical anastomosis of the small intestine to the colon.

enteroenterostomy : surgical anastomosis between two segments of the intestine.

enterolith : a calculus in the intestine.

enterolysis : surgical separation of intestinal adhesions.

enteropexy : surgical fixation of the intestine.

enterorrhaphy : suture of the intestine

enterostomy : the artificial formation of a permanent opening into the intestine through the abdominal wall.

fecal incontinence : loss of voluntary control of defecation.

fecalith : an intestinal concretion formed around a center of fecal material.

fistula : an abnormal passage or communication.

fistulectomy : excision of a fistulous tract.

hemorrhoid : a varicose dilatation of a vein of the superior or inferior hemorrhoidal plexus, resulting from a persistent increase in venous pressure.

hemorrhoidectomy : excision of hemorrhoid.

Hirschsprung's disease : congenital absence of the parasympathetic nerve ganglia in the anorectum or proximal rectum, resulting in the absence of peristalsis in the affected portion of the colon and a consequent massive enlagement of the colon, constipation, and obstruction; called also congenital megacolon.

Hodgkin's disease : a malignant tumor, progressive enlargement of the lymphnodes.

ileitis : inflammation of the ileum, or distal portion of the small intestine.

ileostomy : surgical creation of an opening into the ileum.

imperforate anus : persistence of the anal membrane so that the anus is closed.

intestinal obstruction : any hinderance to the passage of the intestinal contents. causes may be mechanical or neural or both some of the more common mechanical causes are hernia, adhesions of the peritoneum, volvulus, intussuception, malignant or benign tumor, congenital defect, and local inflammation.

intussusception : prolapse of one part of the intestine into the lumen of an immediately adjacent part, causing intestinal obstruction.

jejunectomy : excision of the jejunum.

Jelk's operation : incision of the fibrous tissue around the rectum.

Kraske's operation : an operation for rectal cancer.
Lane's operation : the operation of dividing the ileum near the cecum.
Meckel's diverticulum : a congenital sac or appendage occasionally found in the ileum; a relic of a fetal structure that connects the yolk sac with the intestinal cavity of the embryo.
megacolon, Hirschsprung's disease : abnormally large or dilated colon.
melena : darkening of the feces by blood pigments.
mesopexy : repair of the mesentery.
Mile's operation : abdominoperineal resection for cancer of the lower sigmoid and rectum.
obstipation : intractable constipation.
pilonidal cyst : a hair containing sacrococcygeal dermoid cyst or sinus, often opening at a postnatal dimple.
polyp : a morbid excrescence, or protruding growth, from mucous membrane.
polypectomy : surgical removal of polyp.
proctectomy : excision of the rectum.
proctitis : inflammation of the rectum.
proctopexy : fixation of the rectum.
proctoplasty : plastic repair of the rectum and anus.
proctoscopy : inspection of the rectum with a proctoscope.
proctostomy : surgical creation of a permanent artificial opening from the body surface into the rectum.
prolapse of the rectum : protrusion of the rectal mucous membrane through the anus.
pruritus ani : intense chronic itching in the anal region.
rectocele : hernial protrusion of part of the rectum into the vagina.
steatorrhea : excessive fat in the feces due to a malabsorption syndrome caused by disease, of the intestinal mucosa or pancreatic enzyme deficiency.
tenesmus : ineffectual and painful straining at stool or in urinating.

volvulus : torsion of a loop of intestine, causing obstruction with or without strangulation.

Ⅳ. Liver, pancreas and biliary system

1. Word root

bilirubin/o	bilirubin
celi/o	abdomen
cholangi/o	bile vessel
chol/e, chol/o, bil/i	bile
cholecyst/o	gall bladder
choledoch/o	common bile duct
cirrh/o	hardening
glyc/o, gluc/o	glucose
hepat/o	liver
lapar/o	abdominal wall
lip/o, steat/o	fat
pancreat/o	pancreas
peritone/o	peritoneum

2. Anatomical terms

ampulla of vater	mesocolon
common bile duct	mesoappendix
cystic duct	omentum
gallbladder	pancreas
hepatic duct	pancreatic duct of wirsung
islets of Langerhans	peritoneum
liver	sphincter of Oddi
mesentery	

3. Medical terms

abscess : a localized collection of pus in a cavity formed by the disintergration of tissue.

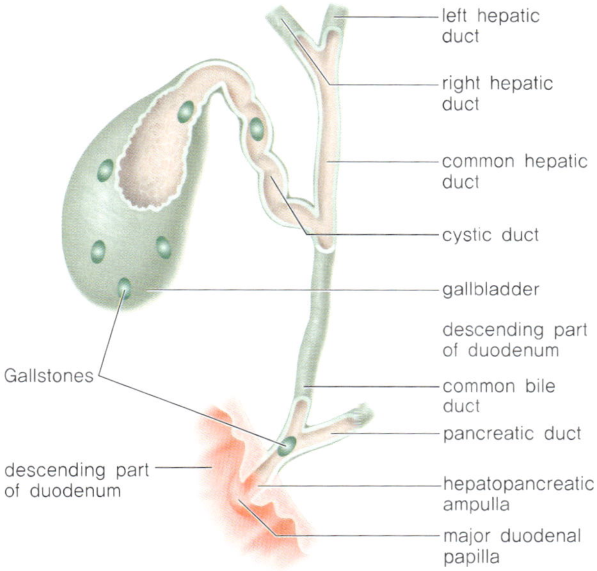

그림 3-8. Gallstone

ascites : abnormal accumulation of serous(edematous) fluid within the peritoneal cavity.

celiotomy : incision into the abdominal cavity.

cholangiography : X-ray examination of the bile ducts, using a radiopaque dye as a contrast medium. In the intravenous method, the dye is administered intravenously and is excreted by the liver into the bile ducts.

cholangitis : inflammation of a bile duct.

cholecystectomy : excision of the gallbladder.

cholecystitis : inflammation of gallbladder, acute or chronic.

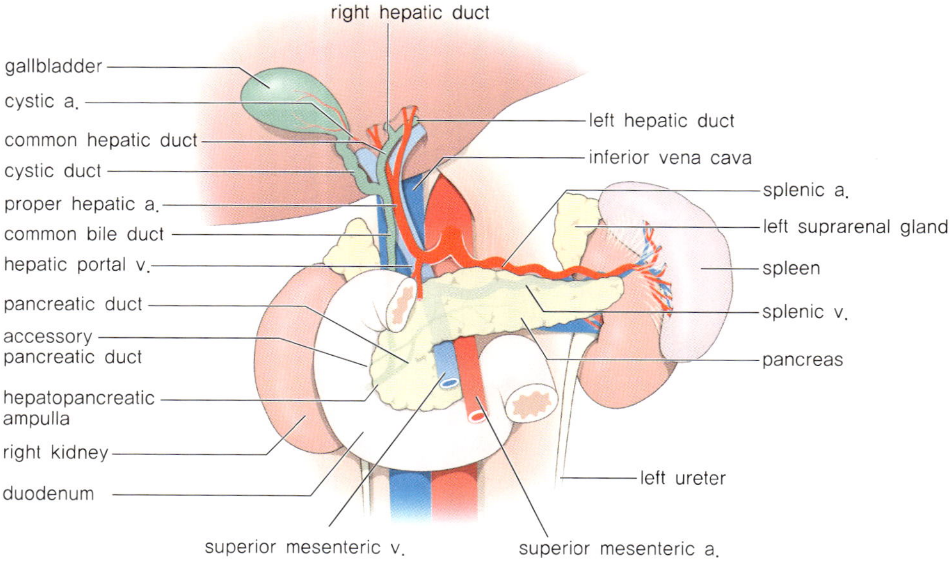

그림 3-9. The pancreas in relation to the livers gallbladder and duodenum

cholecystoduodenostomy : surgical anastomosis of the gallbladder and the duodenum.

cholecystogastrostomy : surgical anastomosis between the gallbladder and the stomach.

cholecystography : roentgenography of the gallbladder, using a radiopaque dye as contrast medium.

cholecystopexy : fixation of the gallbladder.

cholecystostomy : the creation of an opening into the gallbladder for drainage.

cholecystotomy : incision of the gallbladder.

choledochitis : inflammation of the common bile duct.

choledocholithiasis : calculi in the common bile duct.

choledocholithotomy : incision into the common bile duct for removal of stone.

choledochotomy : incision into the common bile duct.

cholelithiasis : the presence or formation of gallstones.

cholelithotripsy : the crushing of gallstones.

cholestasis : stoppage of the flow of bile.

cirrhosis : a liver disease characterized pathologically by loss of replacement of necrotic parenchymal tissue with fibrous bands of connective tissue which eventually constrict and partition the organ into irregular nodules.

coma : a state of unconsciousness from which the patient cannot be aroused, even by powerful stimulation.

diabetes mellitus : a broadly applied term used to denote a complex group of syndromes that have in common a disturbance in the oxidation and utilization of glucose, which is secondary to a malfunction of the beta cells of the pancreas, whose function is the production and release of insulin.

empyema : accumulation of pus in a body cavity.

endoscopy : visual inspection of any cavity of the body by means of an endoscope.

glycosuria : the presence of glucose in the urine.

hemoperitoneum : an effusion of blood in the peritoneal cavity.

hepatectomy : excision of the entire or of a portion of the liver.

hepatic abscess : an abscess of the liver.

hepatic coma : coma accompanying hepatic encephalopathy.

hepatitis : inflammation of the liver.

hepatocellular jaundice : jaundice caused by injury to or disease of the liver cells.

hepatolith : a gallstone, especially one within the liver.

hepatomegaly : enlargement of liver.

hepatorrhaphy : suture of the liver.

hernia : the abnormal protrusion of part of an organ or tissue through the structures normally containing it.

herniorrhaphy : surgical repair of hernia, with suture of the abdominal wall.

hyperglycemia : abnormally in creased content of sugar in the blood.

hypoglycemia : abnormally diminished content of glucose in the blood.

jaundice : yellowness of skin, sclerae, mucous membranes and excretions due to hyperbilirubinemia and deposition of bile pigments. Called also icterus.

laparoscopy : examination of the abdomen by means of a laparoscope.

laparotomy : incision through the flank or, more generally, through any part of the abdominal wall.

liver biopsy : removal and examination usually microscopic tissue from the living body.

mesenteritis : inflammation of the mesentery.

obstructive jaundice : due to an impediment to the flow of the bile from the liver cells to the duodenum.

pancreatalgia : pain in the pancreas.

pancreatectomy : excision of the pancreas.

pancreatic lithiasis : the presence of calculi in the pancreas.

pancreatic pseudocyst : an encapsulated collection of pancreatic juice and cellular debris that has escaped from the pancreas, the wall being formed by inflammatory fibrosis of serosal surfaces of adjacent organs.

pancreatitis : inflammation of the pancreas, which is due to autodigestion of panereatic tissue by its own enzymes.

peritoneal abscess : collection of inflammatory exudate in peritonitis.

peritoneocentesis : puncture of the peritoneal cavity with a needle for the purpose of obtaining.

peritonitis : inflammation of the peritoneum.

pneumoperitonium : the presence of gas in the peritoneal cavity.

pseudocyst : an abnormal or dilated space resembling a cyst but not lined by epithelium as is a true cyst.

tympanites : drumlike distention of the abdomen due to air or gas in the intestine or peritoneal cavity, called also tympanism.

viral hepatitis : an acute infectious hepatitis caused by one of at least two different viral strains : hepatitis A virus and hepatitis B virus. Type A hepatitis was formerly called infectious hepatitis, epidemic hepatitis and acute catarrhal jaundice. Type B hepatitis was formerly called serum hepatitis, hemologous serum jaundice and long incubation period hepatitis.

Whipple's operation : radical pancreatoduodenectomy.

Chapter 4 URINARY SYSTEM

I. Urinary organs and structure

kidneys : two, lie behind the abdominal organs against muscles of the back(retroperitoneal) and are held in place by fat. The parts of the kidney include the following :

cortex : outer layer.

medulla : inner portion.

nephrons : kidney cells and capillaries. The glomerulus, Bowmans capsule, and renal collecting tubule are all parts of the nephrons. The nephrons are the parenchyma(functioning parts) of the kidney.

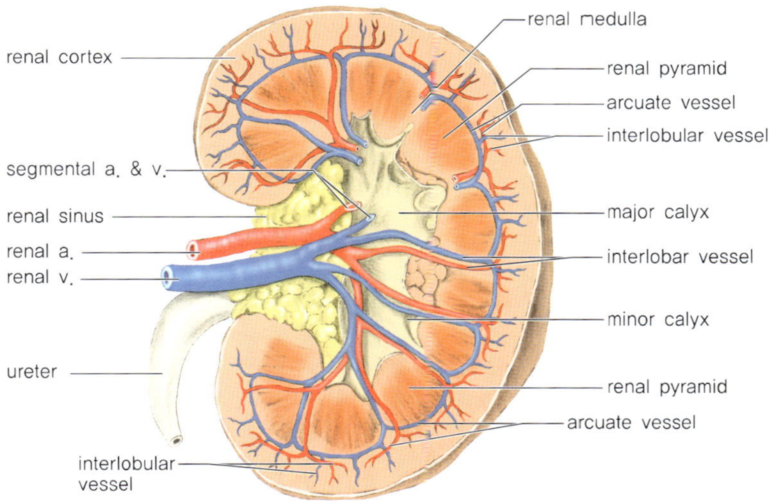

그림 4-1. The kidney

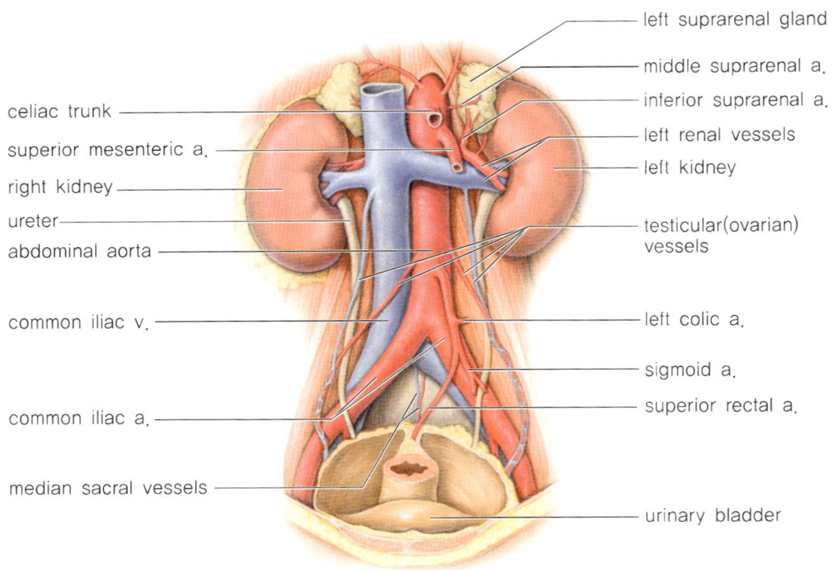

그림 4-2. Organs of the urinary system

renal pelvis : the wide, upper end of the ureter(lies inside kidney).

ureters : narrow tubes lined with mucous membrane. Urine passes from the kidneys, through the renal pelvis, and is moved through the ureters by peristalsis.

urethra : in female-narrow short tube from bladder to exterior ; in male-narrow long tube, carries urine and seminal fluid to exterior.

urinary bladder : lined with mucous membrane ; urine collects here, and bladder expands to hold urine.

urinary meatus : opening of the urethra to exterior.

Ⅱ. Function of the system

to filter the blood. Urine is formed by the nephrons.

1. Water and substances in solution are removed from blood.
2. Essential water and substances are reabsorbed.
3. Some water and dissolved substances are excreted to regulate reaction of the blood. Reaction of blood(pH) normally is slightly alkaline.

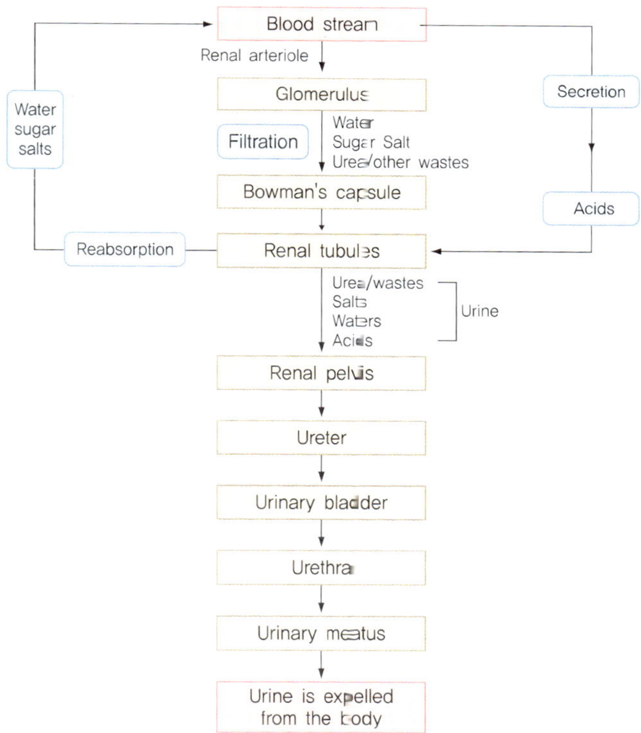

그림 4-3. Flow diagram of the process of forming and expelling process

1. Word root

cortic/o	cortex
cyst/o, vesic/o	urinary bladder
glomerul/o	glomerulus
medull/o	medulla
nephr/o, ren/o	kidney
pyel/o	renal pelvis
ur/o	urine
ure/o, azot/o	urea
ureter/o	reter
urethr/o	rethra
uric/o	uric acid
vesicul/o, vesic/o, cyst/o	urinary bladder

2. Anatomical terms

Bowmans capsule	renal medulla
calyx	renal pelvis
hilum, hilus of kidney	renal pyramid
infundibulum	trigone
nephron	tubules
renal cortex	urethra
renal glomerulus	

3. Medical terms

anuria : complete suppression of urine formation by the kidney.

azotemia : the presence of nitrogen-containing compounds in the blood.

cyctitis : inflammation of the urinary bladder.

cystoceles : herniation of the urinary bladder into the vagina.

cystoscopy : direct visual examination of the urinary tract with a cystoscope.

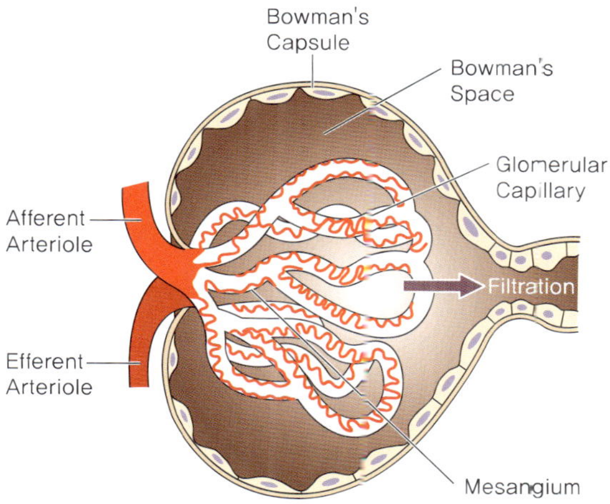

그림 4-4. Glomerulus and Bowman's capsule

duplication of ureters : partial or complete duplication of one or both ureters.

dysuria : difficult urgency.

edema : an abnormal accumulation of fluid.

enuresis : involuntary discharge of urine, usually referring to involuntary discharge of urine during sleep at night ; bed wetting.

frequency of urination : urination at short intervals without increase in daily volume of urinary output, due to reduced bladder capacity.

glomerulonephritis : a variety of nephritis characterized by inflammation of the capillary loops in the glomeruli of the kidney.

glomerulosclerosis : arteriolar nephrosclerosis.

hydronephrosis : distension of the renal pelvis and calices with urine.

hydroureter : ureteral overdistention caused by the obstruction.

hypernephroma : adenocarcinoma of the renal cortex.

incontinence of urine : inability to control excretory functions.

intravenous pyelography : roentgenography of the kidney and ureter after injection of a contrast medium introduced by the intravenous method.

malignant nephroangiosclerosis : renal arteriolar necrosis associated with hypertention.

measurement of renal function : evaluating the severity of renal disease and in following its progess.

nephroblastoma : a rapidly developing malignant mixed tumor of the kidneys, made up of embryonal elements, and occurring chiefly in children before the fifth year; called also Wilms tumor.

nephrocalcinosis : deposition of calcium phosphate in the renal tubules, resulting in renal insufficiency.

nephrolithotomy : incision of kidney for removal of calculi.

nephrectomy : surgical removal of a kidney.

nephritis : inflammation of the kidney; a focal or diffuse proliferative of destructive disease that may involve the glomerulus, tubule, or interstitial renal tissue ; called also Brights disease.

nephrolithiasis : a condition marked by the presence of renal calculi.

nephrolysis : freeing of a kidney from adhesions.

nephropexy : surgical fixation of a floating or hypermobile kidney(nephroptosis).

nephroptosis : downward displacement of a kidney.

nephrosis : any kidney disease, especially disease marked by purely degenerative lesions of the renal tubules; called also nephrotic syndrome.

nephrotomy : incision of the kidney.

nocturia : excessive urination at night.

pneumaturia : the presence of air or gas in the urine.

polyuria : excessive excretion of urine.

prostatitis : inflammation of the prostate.

proteinuria : an excess of serum proteins in the urine.

pyelitis : inflammation of the renal pelvis.

pyelolithotomy : incision of the renal pelvis for removal of calculi.

pyelonephritis : inflammation of the kidney and renal pelvis.

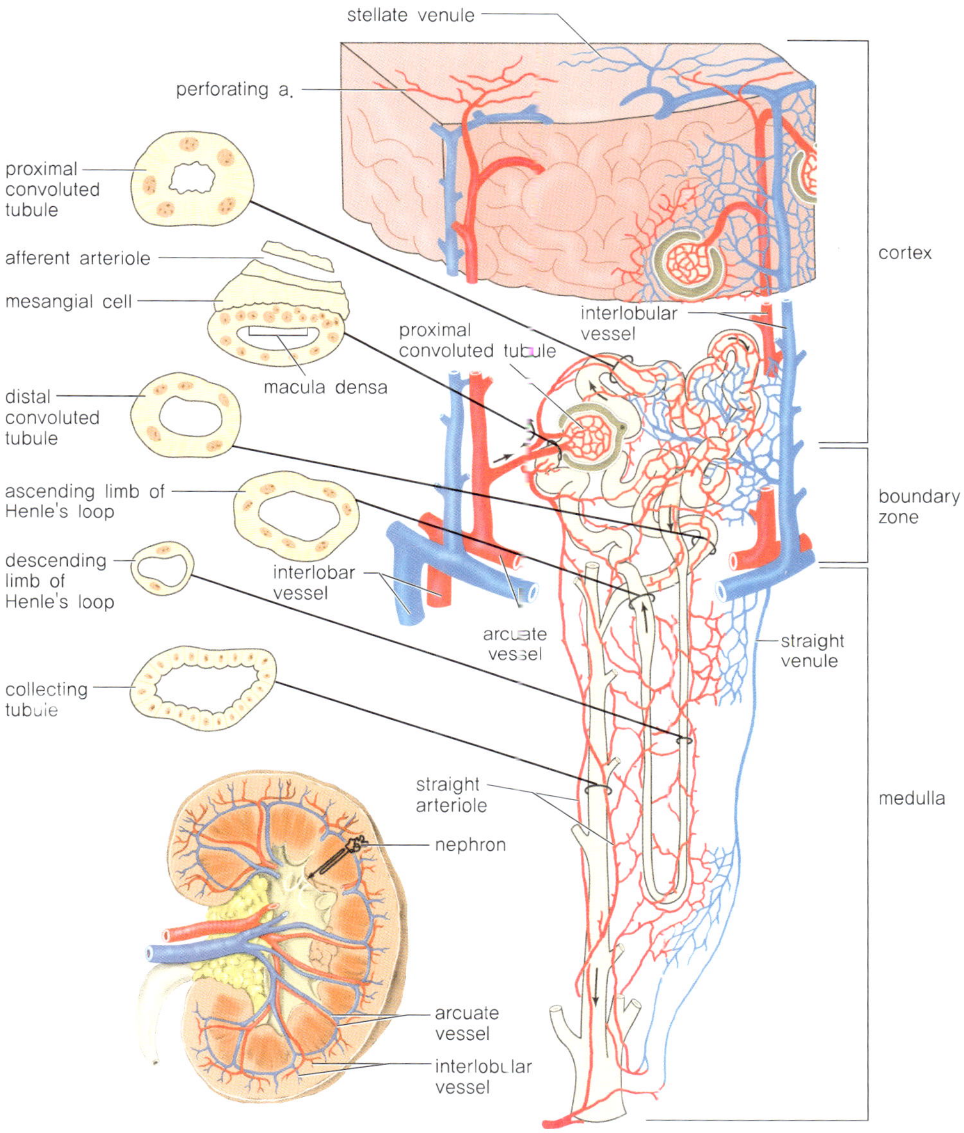

그림 4-5. Nephrons (a) Juxtamedullary nephron (b) Cortical nephron

pyuria : pus in the urine.

renal abscess : a focal, suppurative lesion of the renal parenchyma tissues.

renal failure : inability of the kidney to maintain normal function.

renal infarction : ischemic necrosis of renal tissue.

renal tuberculosis : tuberculosis of the kidney.

renovascular hypertention : elevation of systemic BP caused by partial or complete occlution of renal arteries.

retention of urine : accumulation of urine within the bladder because of inability to urinate.

retrograde pyelography : roentgenography of the kidney and ureter after introduction of the contrast medium by way of ureteral catheters.

retrograde urethrography : radiography of the urethra after the injection of an contrast medium through the urethra.

stress incontinence : partial incompetence of the urinary spincter.

uremia : an excess in the blood of urea, creatinine, and other nitrogenous end products of protein and amino acid metabolism; more correctly referred to as azotemia.

ureteral obstruction, stenosis : obstrution and stricture of the ureter.

ureterocele : bulging of the lower end of the ureter into the bladder.

ureterostenosis : stricture of the ureter.

urethritis : inflammation of the urethra.

urethrocele : prolapse of the female urethra through the urinary meatus.

urethral obstrution : obstustion in the urethra.

urinalysis : physical, chemical, or microscopic analysis or examination of urine.

urinary calculus : a calculus of the urinary tract.

vesical tenesmus : ineffectual and painful straining in urinating.

vesicoureteral reflux : reflux of urine from the bladder into the ureter.

voiding cystourethrography : radiography of the urinary bladder and urethra in which the radiography made before, during and after voiding.

Wilm's tumor : a rapidly developing malignant mixed tumor of the kidneys, made up of embryonal elements, and occurring chiefly in children before the fifth year; called also embryonal carcinosarcoma and nephroblastoma.

Chapter 5

MALE REPRODUCTIVE SYSTEM

I. Male reproductive (genital) organs

testes(testis) : also called testicles ; sex glands, located in scrotum. They form spermatozoa(sex cells) and secrete the hormone testosterone.

ducts

epididymis : at top of each testis ; spermatozoa are stored in these ducts.

vasdeferens : ductus deferens ; excretory duct of the testis.

seminal duct : excretory duct of the seminal vesicle.

ejaculatory duct : canal formed by union of ductus (vas) deferens and the excretory duct of the seminal vesicle.

urethra : opening for sperm and urine passage.

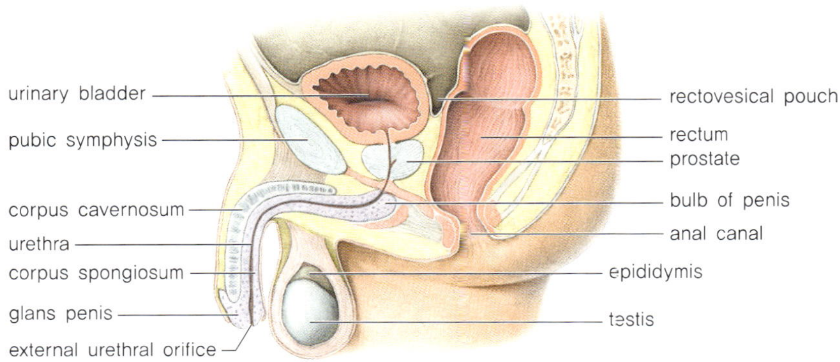

그림 5-1. Median sagittal section of the male pelvis with a portion of the left pubic bone attached to illustrate the path of the ductus deferens.

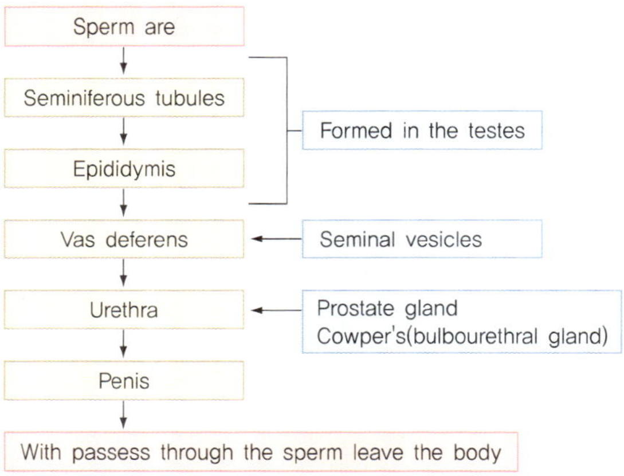

그림 5-2. The passaage of sperm from the seminiferous tubules in the testes to the outside of the body

accessory glands : secrete alkaline secretions that together with sperm make up seminal fluid.

prostate gland : surrounds urethra ; secretes alkaline fluid that forms part of semen. Tends to enlarge in older men and may block flow of urine.

external genitalia : scrotum and penis.

Ⅱ. Function of the system

1. Word root

andr/o	male
balan/o	glans penis
crypt/o	hidden
epididym/o	epididymis
orch/o, orchid/o, orchi/o	testis
prostat/o	prostate gland
sperm/o, spermat/o	spermatozoa
test/o	testis
vas/o	vessel, duct
vesicul/o	seminal vesicles

2. Anatomical terms

epididymis	seminal vesicles
glans penis	sperm, spermatozoon
penis	spermatic cord
prosta	tetestis
scrotum	vas deferens
semen	

3. Medical terms

anorchism : congenital absence of one or both testes.

azoospermia : absence of spermatozoa in the semen, or failure of formation of spermatozoa.

balanitis : inflammation of the glans penis.

balanoplasty : plastic surgery of the glans penis.

benign prostatic hypertrophy : enlargement of the prostate. Because of its position around the urethra, enlargement of the prostate quickly interferes with the normal passage of urine from the bladder.

castration : bilateral orchiectomy and oophorectomy.

chancre : in the primary lesion of syphilis, occurring at the site of entry of the infection, called also hard, hunterian, or true chancre.

chancroid : a soft nonsyphilitic veneral sore caused by Haemophilus Ducreyi.

circumcision : surgical removal of all or part of the foreskin, or prepuce, of the penis.

cryptorchism : failure of one of both of the testes to descend into the scrotum.

cystectomy : excision or resection of the urinary bladder.

cystitis : inflammation of the urinary bladder.

cystocele : herniation of the urinary bladder into the vagina.

cystoscopy : examination of the bladder by means of a cystoscope, a hollow metal tube that is introduced into the urinary meatus and passed through the urethra and into the bladder.

epididymectomy : excision of the epididymis.

epididymitis : inflammation of the epididymis. Nonspecific epididymitis may result from an infection in the urinary tract, especially in the prostate.

epididymoorchitis : inflammation of the epididymis and testis.

epispadias : congenital absence of the upper wall of the urethra, the urethral opening being anywhere on the drosum of the penis, and manifested as a groove or cleft without a covering.

fistulectomy : excision of fistulous tract.

funiculitis : inflammation of the spermatic cord.

gonorrhea : an acute infecious disease of the epithelium of the genital tract; caused by Neisseria gonorrhoeae.

hydrocele : a collection of fluid in the tunica vaginalis of the testide.

hydroureter : distention of the ureter with fluid, due to obstruction.

hypergonadism : abnormally inceased functional activity of the gonads.

hypospadias : a developmental anomaly in the male in which the urethra opens on the under side of the penis or on the perineum.

inguinal hernia : hernia into the inguinal canal.

male hypogonadism : abnormally decreased functional activity of the gonads.

meatotomy : incision of the urinary meatus in order to enlarge it.

oligospermia : deficiency of spermatozoa in the semen.

orchiectomy : excision of one or both testes.

orchiopexy : surgical fixation of an undescended testis in the scrotum.

Peyronie's disease : dysplasia of the covernous sheaths in the penis.

phimosis : constriction of the orifice of the prepuce so that it cannot be drawn back over the glans.

polycystic kidney disease : a hereditary disease in which there is a massive enlargement of the kidney accompanied by the formation of cysts.

prostatectomy : surgical removal of the prostate.

prostatitis : inflammation of the prostate

prostatography : the detection of calcareous deposits and, as shown by urinary retention, of prostatic enlargement.

scrotal varicocele : a collection of veins of the pampiniform plexus.

spermatocele : a cystic distention of the epididymis or the rete testis containing spermatozoa.

spermatocelectomy : operative excision of a lesion of the epididymis.

syphilis : a contagious systemic disease caused by the spirochete Treponema pallidum.

ureterectomy : excision of a ureter.

ureteritis : inflammation of the ureter.

ureterocolostomy : anastomosis of a ureter to the colon.

ureteroileostomy : anastomosis of the ureters to an isolated loop of the ileum, drained through a stoma on the abdominal wall.

ureterolithiasis : formation of a calculus in the ureter.

ureterolithotomy : incision of a ureter for removal of calculus.

ureteroneocystostomy : surgical transplantation of a ureter to a different site in the bladder ; ureterocystostomy.

urethritis : inflammation of the urethra.

urethroplasty : plastic repair of the urethra.

varicocele : varicosity of the pampiniform plexus of the spermatic cord, forming scrotal swelling that feels like a bag of worms.

varicocelectomy : the excision of a part of the scrotum and the enlarged veins for varicocele.

vasectomy : excision of the vas deferens, or a portion of it; bilateral vasectomy results in sterility.

vasoligation : ligation of the vas ductus deferens.

vasovasostomy : anastomosis of the ends of the severed vas ductus deferens.

vesicorectal fistula : any abnormal, tubelike passage between the bladder and the rectum.

vesicovaginal fistula : any abnormal, tubelike passage between the bladder and the vagina.

Chapter

6 FEMALE REPRODUCTIVE SYSTEM

Ⅰ. Female reproductive (genital) organs

ovaries : sex glands, located in pelvis. They form ova(ovum))sex cells. Ovulation-ovum leaves ovary.

Follicles secrete hormones : estrogens and progesterones.

ducts : fallopian tubes, where fertilization occurs ; fringe-like distal parts called fimbria.

uterus : top part called the fundus ; the neck(cervix) opens into the vagina.

vagina : birth canal ; vaginal introitus, entrance to vagina.

Bartholins glands : accessory mucous glands.

external genitals : organs of generation vulva or pudendum(labia majora and minora).

breasts : lactation controlled by hormones.

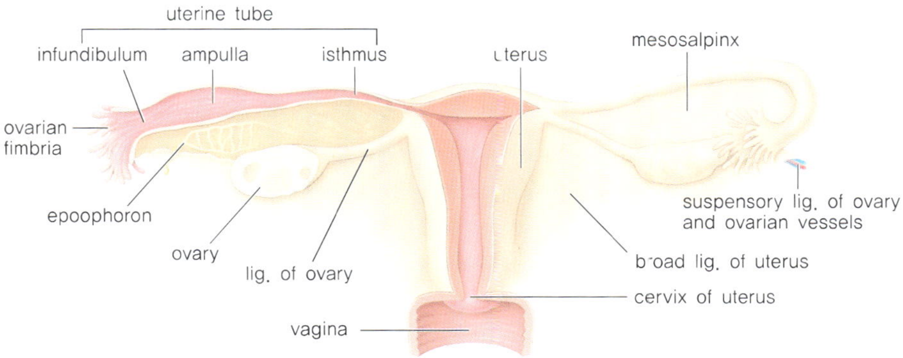

그림 6-1. Structures of the female reproductive system as seen from behind. The posterior walls of the vagina, the left side of the uterus, and the left uterine tube have been removed, as has the entire left broad ligament.

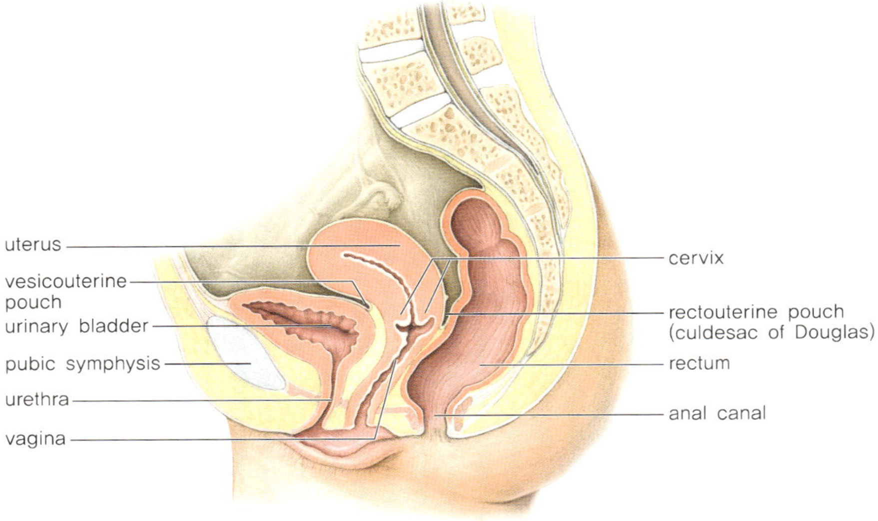

그림 6-2. Female organs of reproduction seen in sagittal section

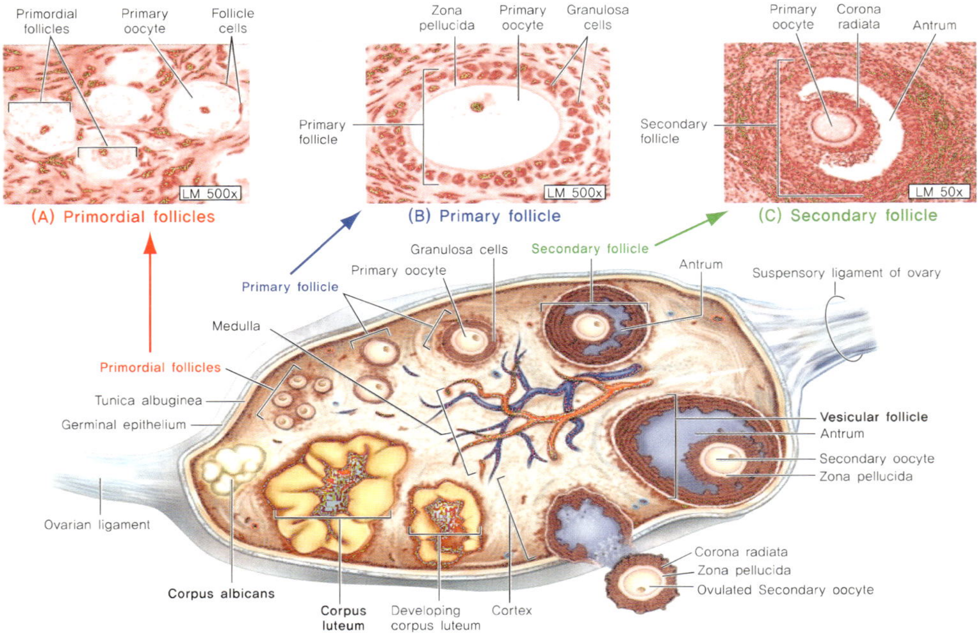

그림 6-3. Parts of the ovary seen in sectional view. The arrows indicate the sequence of developmental stages that occur as part of the ovarian cycle.

Ⅱ. Function of the system

1. Word root

amni/o	amnion
cervic/o, trachel/o	cervix
chori/o	chorion
colp/o, vagin/o	vagina
episi/o, pudend/o, vulv/o	vulva
gravid/o	regnancy
gynec/o, gyn/o	female
hyster/o, metr/o, uter/o	uterus
lact/o	milk
mamm/o, mast/o	breast
men/o	menstruation
oo/o, ov/o	egg
ovari/o, oophor/o	ovary
perine/o	erineum
salping/o	fallopian tubes
thel/o	nipple
vulv/o, episi/o	vulva

2. Anatomical terms

(1) Vulva

Bartholin's gland	perineum
clitoris	prepuce
hymen	Skenes gland
labia majora	vagina
labia minora	vestibule
mons pubis	vulva
paraurethral duct	vulvovaginal gland

(2) Uterus

broad ligament	parametrium
cervix uteri	rectouterine pouch
corpus uteri	round ligament
endometrium	serosa
external os	uterine cavity
fundus uteri	uterovesical pouch
internal os	uterus
myometrium	

(3) Ovary

adnexa uteri	infundibulum
corpus albicans	menstruation
corpus luteum	ovary
fallopian tube	ovulation
fimbria	ovum
graafian follicle	primordial follicle

(4) Breast

alveolus tissue	lobe of mammary gland
areola	mammary duct
breast	mammary gland
lactiferous dust	

3. Medical terms

abdominal hysterectomy : that performed through the abdominal wall.

abortion : the premature explusion from the uterus of the products of conceptions.

adenomyosis : the benign invasion of endometrium into the myometrium.

amenorrhea : absence of the menses.

amniocentesis : surgical tansabdominal perforation of the uterus, to obtain amniotic fluid.

amniotomy : deliberate rupture of the fetal membranes.

Bartholin's adenitis : inflammation of the bartholin gland.

candidiasis : infection by candida albicans, most commonly involving the skin, oral mucosa(thrush), respiratory tract, and vagina; called also moniliasis.

carcinoma : a malignant new growth made up of epithelial cells tending to infiltrate surrounding tissues and to give rise to metastasis.

cervical polyp : inflammatory tumor protruded from mucous membranes of the uterine cervix.

cervicectomy : excision of the cervix uteri.

cervicitis : inflammation of the cervix uteri.

colpitis : inflammation of the vaginal mucosa; called also vaginitis.

condyloma : an elevated wartlike lesion of the skin.

condyloma acuminatum : a small, pointed papilloma of viral origin, usually occurring on the skin or mucous surfaces of the external genitalia or perianal region.

cryotherapy : the therapeutic use of cold.

dilatation & curettage : expanding of the ostium uteri to permit scraping of the walls the uterus.

dysmenorrhea : painful menstruation.

dystocia : abnormal labor or childbirth.

eclampsia : coma and or convulsive seizures between the 20th week of pregnancy.

ectopic pregnancy : pregnancy in which implantation occurs outside the endometrium and endometrial cavity.

endometrial hyperplasia : abnormal overgrowth of the endometrium.

endometriosis : a condition in which tissue more of less perfectly resembling the uterine mucous membrane occurs aberrantly in various locations in the pelvic cavity.

endometritis : inflammation of the endometrium.

erosion of cervix : destruction of the squamous epithelium of the vaginal portion of the cervix, due to irritation; the eroded area is covered by columnar epithelium.

fetus : the unborn offspring before the birth.

Goodell's sign : If the woman's cervix uteri is soft, she is pregnant.

gynecomastia : hypertrophy in the male breast.

hirsutism : abnormal hairness in women.

hydramnios : excessive amount of amniotic fluid.

hydrocolpos : a collection of watery fluid in the vagina.

hydrosalpinx : a collection of watery fluid in a uterine tube, occurring as the end stage of pyosalpinx.

hyperemesis grabidarum : malignant nausea and vomiting in the pregnant women.

hypermenorrhea : excessive uterine bleeding occuring at regular intervals.

hypomenorrhea : uterine bleeding of less than the normal account.

hysterectomy : surgical removal of the uterus.

hysteropexy : fixation of a displaced uterus by surgery.

hysterosalpingography : roentgenography of the uterus and uterine tubes after the injection of opaque material.

immature infant : one weighing 500 to 999 grams at birth, usually before the twenty eighth week of gestation.

imperforate hymen : abnormally closed hymen.

induced abortion : abortion brought on intentionally.

induced labor : labor brought on by mechanical or other extraneous.

infertility : the inability to conceive and produce viable offspring.

labor : the act or process of giving birth to a child.

laparoscopy : examination of the interior of the abdomen by means of a laparoscope.

leukorrhea : a whitish, viscid discharge from the vagina and uterine cavity.

mast-adenitis, mastitis : inflammation of the mammary gland.

mastalgia : pain in the mammary gland.

mastectomy : excision of the breast.

meconium : mucilaginous material in the intestine of the full term fetus.

Meigs's syndrome : ascites and hydrothorax associated with ovarian fibroma.

menarche : establishment or beginning of the menstrual function.

menopause : the span of time during which the menstrual cycle wanes and gradually stops; called also climacteric.

menorrhagia : excessive menstruation.

metrorrhagia : uterine bleeding, usually of normal amount, occurring at completely irregular intervals, the period of flow sometimes being prolonged.

myoma : a tumor formed of muscle tissue.

myoma uteri : a benign tumor of the smooth muscle fibers of the uterus; called also myoma of uterus.

radical hysterectomy : excision of the uterus, upper vagina, and parametrium.

retroflexion of uterus : the bending backward of the body of the uterus upon the cervix.

retroversion of uterus : the tipping backward of an uterus.

oligomenorrhea : abnormally infrequent menstruation.

oophorectomy : excision of one or both ovaries; called also ovariectomy.

oophoritis : inflammation of an ovary.

oophorocystectomy : excision of an ovarian cyst.

oophoropexy : fixation of a displaced ovary by surgery.

oophorosalpingectomy : surgical removal of a uterine tube and ovary.

Paget's disease of the breast : an inflammatory cancerous affection of the areola and nipple.

palpation : the act of the feeling with the hand.

Papanicolaou test : examines exfoliated cells to detect malignant and premalignant condition of the female genital tract.

parametritis : inflammation of the parametrium.

pelvic inflammatory disease : include infection of the cervix(cervicitis), the uterus(endometritis), or the ovaries(oophoritis) as well.

pelvimetry : the measurement of the dimensions and capacity of the pelvis.

perineorrhaphy : suture of the oerineum.

placenta accreta : abnormal adherence of part or all of the placenta to the uterine wall.

placenta previa : implantation of the placenta over or near the internal os of the cervix.

placentitis : inflammation of the placenta.

placentography : radiological visualization of the placenta after the inje-ction of a contrast medium.

polyp : any growth or mass protruding from a mucous membrane.

preeclampsia : development of hypertension, albuminuria, or edema between the 20th week of pregnancy.

premature infant : born after the twenty seventh week and before full term, weighing 1000 to 2499 grams at birth.

premature separation of placenta : premature separation of a normally implanted placenta from the uterus.

prolapse of uterus : downward displacement of the uterus so that the cervix is within the vaginal orifice(first-degree prolapse), the cervix is outside the orifice(second-degree prolapse), or the entire uterus is outside the orifice(third-degree prolapse).

puerperal infection : infection of genital tract occuring after the postpartum.

pyosalpinx : a collection of pus in an oviduct.

quickening : the first recognizable movements of the fetus.

salpingectomy : excision of a uterine tube.

salpingitis : inflammation of a uterine tube.

salpingostomy : surgical restoration of the patency of a uterine tube.

spontaneous abortion : abortion occuring naturally.

spontaneous labor : labor in which no artificial air is required.

sterility : the state of being sterile.

still-birth : the delivery of a dead child.

subtotal hysterectomy : that in which the cervix is left in place.

total hysterectomy : that in which the uterus and cervix are completely excised.

toxemia of pregnancy : a group of pathogenic conditions occuring in pregnant women.

trichomoniasis : a sexually transmitted disease caused by Trichomanas vaginalis. In females, vaginal or urethral infections may be asymptomatic or may produce itching or burning, dysuria, and vaginal urethral discharges.

uterine leiomyoma : benign tumor of the uterus derived from smooth muscle.

ultrasonography : an imaging technic in differentiating cystic from solid breast masses.

vaginal hysterectomy : that performed through the vagina.

vaginectomy, colpectomy : excision of the vagina.

vermix caseosa : an unctuous substance covers the skin of the fetus.

vulva dermatitis : dermatitis of vulva.

vulvovaginitis : inflammation of the vulva and vagina.

Wertheim's operation : radical hysterectomy.

xeroradiography(soft tissue X-ray) : a dry, totally photoelectric process for recording X-ray images. Using metal plates coated with a semiconductor.

Chapter 7

NERVOUS SYSTEM

I. Central nervous system(cns)

The CNS coordinates and controls all of the bodys activities and, together with the endocrine system, helps to maintain homeostasis.

brain

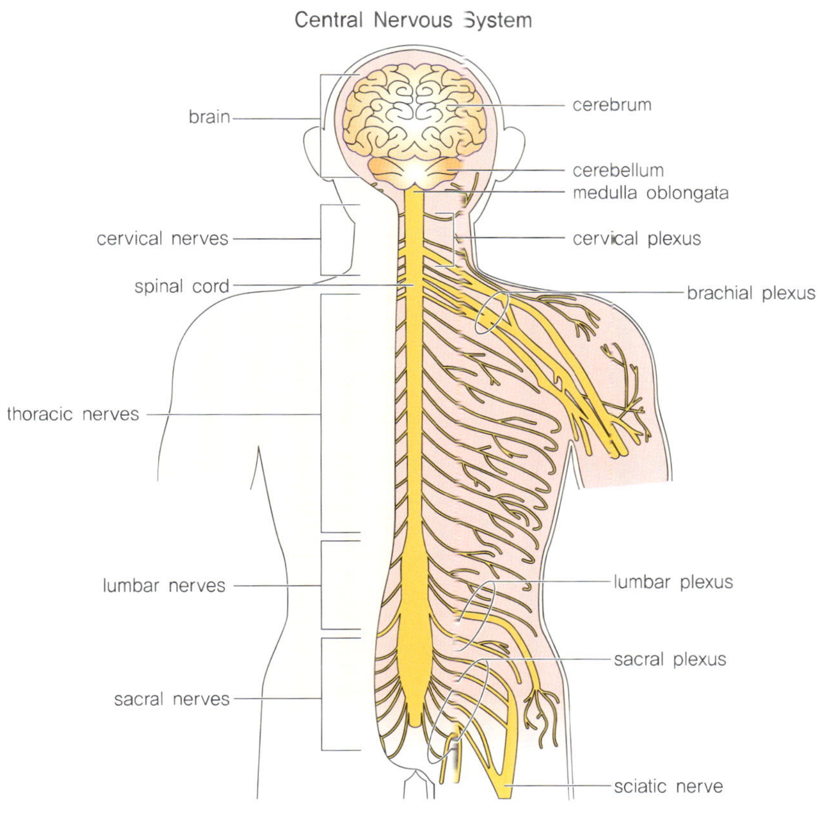

그림 7-1. The central nervous system consition of the brain and the spinal cord

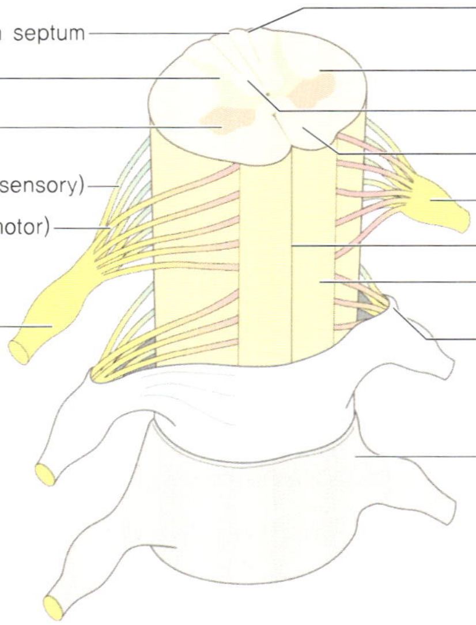

그림 7-2. The meninges that surround the spinal cord

cerebrum : (largest part) ; lobes : frontal, parietal, temporal, and occipital ; function : consciousness, mental processes, sensations, emotions and voluntary movement.

cerebellum : occupies posterior cranial fossa(shallow depression) behind brain stem ; function : maintains equilibrium, normal postures, coordination.

brain stem : pons and medulla oblongata. An enlarged extension of the spinal cord. Contains the vital centers : cardiac, vasomotor, and respiratory centers. Function : controls rate and strength of heart beat, constriction and dilatation of blood vessels, and rate and depth of respirations.

spinal cord : lies inside the spinal column(vertebral column) from the occipital bone through the foramen magnum down to the first lumbar vertebra. Function : conducts impulses between the brain and other parts of the body and serves as a center for reflexes.

meninges(singular is meninx) : are membranes that cover the spinal cord and brain.

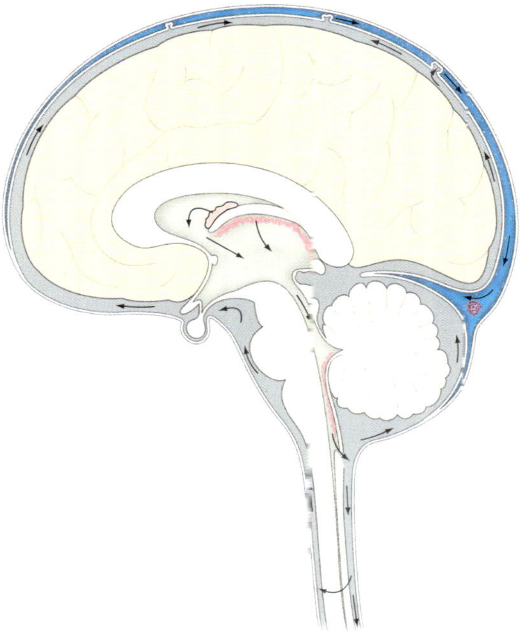

그림 7-3. The location of the cerebrospinal fluid that surrounds the brain and spinal cord. The arrow indicate the direction of the fow of the fluid.

dura mater : tough outer covering.

arachnoid : middle layer.

piameter : internal layer, directly covering brain and cord.

cerebrospinal fluid(CSF) : fluid that circulates around the cord and the brain, in the subarachnoid space.

Ⅱ. Autonomic nervous system (Peripheral nervous system)

cranial nerves : 12 pairs.

1. Olfactory(sense of smell).
2. Optic(vision).
3. Oculomotor(movement of eyes).
4. Trochlear(muscle of eyes).
5. Trigeminal(facial movements).
6. Abducens(eye muscles that turn eye outward).
7. Facial(muscles of face, ears, scalp).
8. Auditory(hearing and equilibrium).
9. Glossopharyngeal(secretion of parotid gland, taste).
10. Pneumogastric, vagus(voice and swallowing).
11. Spinal(neck muscles).
12. Hypoglossal(tongue).

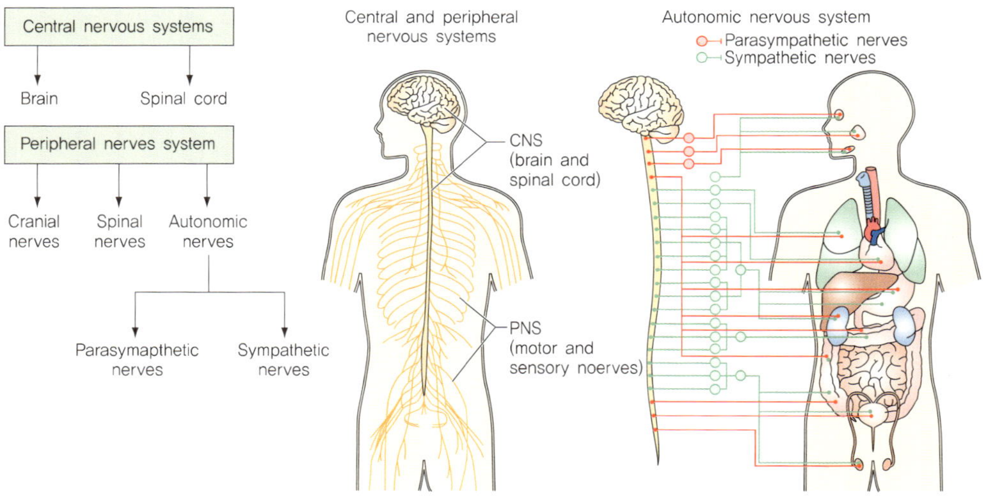

그림 7-4. Divisions of the nervous system

spinal nerves : 31 pairs attached to spinal cord. Numbered according to the section of the spinal column ; for example, C-1 is first cervical, T-8 is eighth thoracic, and so on. Co is the coccyx.

The autonomic nervous system is called involuntary because we do not control it(circulation, for example). It conducts impulses out from the brain stem or spinal cord to smooth muscle, cardiac muscle, and so on. (Autonomic means self-governing.)

plexus : a network of nerves(or blood or lymph vessels) ; Example : solar plexus located behind the stomach. Tabers dictionary lists all of the plexuses in an appendix.

The autonomic nervous system is further divided into two divisions :

sympathetic : (cell bodies originate in thoracolumbar sections T-1 to L-2) assists the body in emergencies, defense, and survival. Adrenergic refers to sympathetic nerve fibers that produce an adrenalin-like substance.

parasympathetic : (cell bodies originate in craniosacral sections) brings the body functions back to normal, after the stressful situation has ended. Cholinergic refers to nerve fibers or agents that produce the effect of acetylcholine to block the action of parasympathetic nerves.

In general, these two divisions have opposing functions ; they are important in maintenance of the bodys homeostatic condition. Following are some examples of their action :

Sympathetic (adrenergic nerves)		Parasympathetic (cholinergic nerves)
Constrict	Cerebral arteries	Dilate
Dilate	Pupils	Constrict
Increased	Metabolic rate	No action
Dilate	Bronchi	Constrict
Constrict	Pulmonary arterioles	Dilate
Rate increased	Heart	Rate decreased
Decreased	Stomach/GI motility	Increased

Nervous System

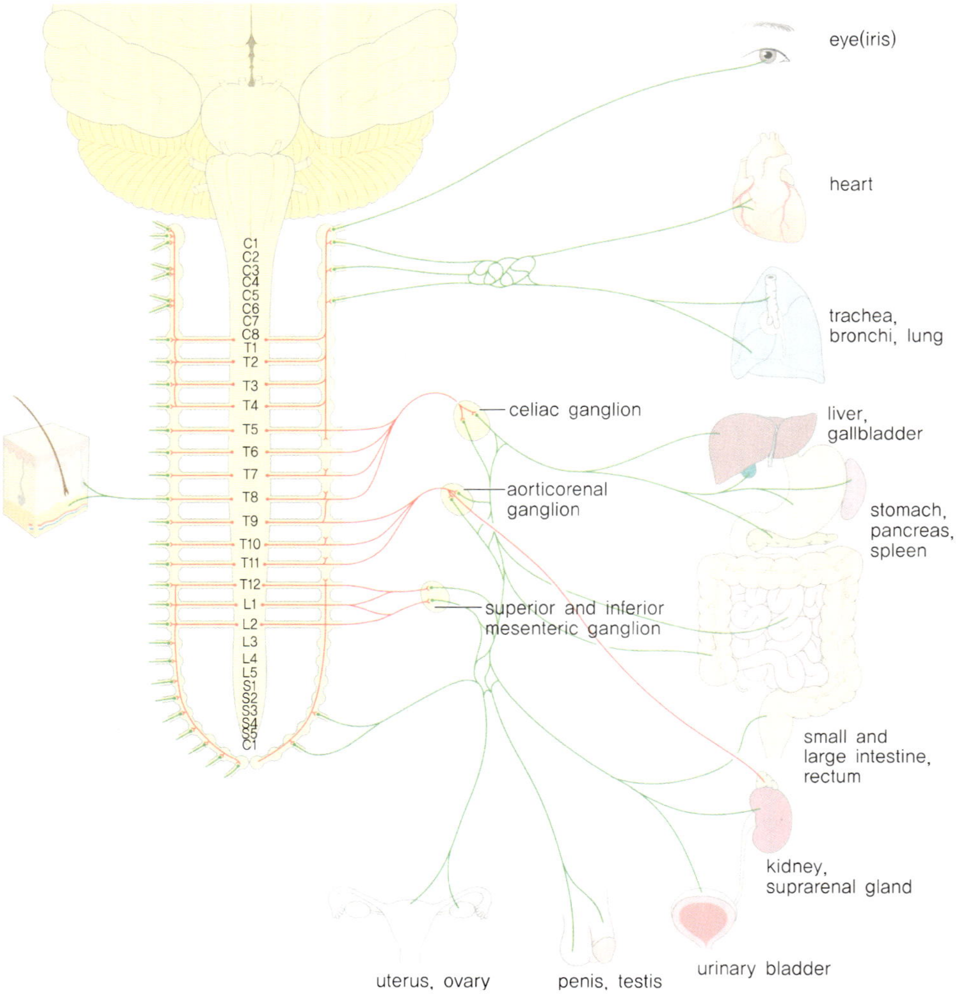

그림 7-5. The sympathetic nervous system

NERVE CELLS (NEURONS) : respond to stimuli(stimulus-response) and special-ize in transmitting impulses. Nervous tissue is extremely delicate and is well protected by bones of the cranium and spinal column. Further protection is provided by the membranes(meninges) and the cerebrospinal fluid.

SPECIALISTS : Patients with neurological disorders or injury to the brain or cord are usually treated by neurologists and neurosurgeons. Other involved specialists are internists, radiologists, psychiatrists, and physiatrists.

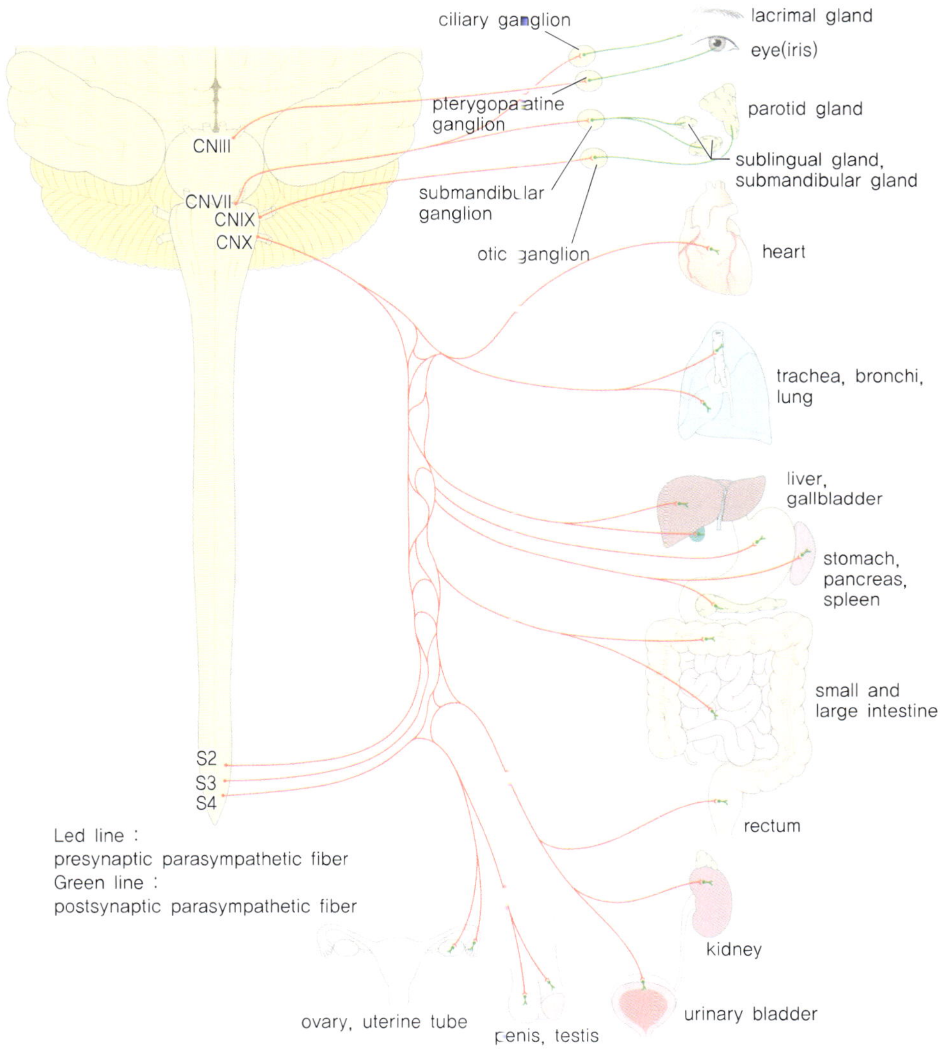

그림 7-6. The parasympathetic nervous system

THE NEUROLOGICAL EXAMINATION

mental status : intellect ; affect(mood or emotional state) ; orientation as to time/place ; disordered thought, such as delusions, hallucinations, illusions ; insight ; consciousness ; language function.

cranial nerves : tested separately for taste, touch, temperature, visual acuity, position sense, and so on.

spinal cord and peripheral nerves

1. Motor function : muscles, adequate strength, quick contraction, prompt relaxation ;flaccid and spastic paralysis.
2. Sensory function : touch, pain, position, vibration.
3. Complex functions : involved movement, coordination, reflexes (including Babinski), balance (Romberg).

Ⅲ. Function of the system

1. Word root

arachn/o	arachnoid membrane
cerebell/o	cerebellum
cerebr/o	brain, cerebrum
chord/o	cord, chord
dur/o	dura, dura mater
encephal/o	brain
ganglio/o	ganglion
gli/o	gluey substance neuroglia
gyr/o	gyrus
mening/o	meninges
myel/o	spinal cord
neur/o	nerve
plex/o	plexus, network
poli/o	gray matter
pont/o	pons
thalam/o	thalamus
ventricul/o	ventricle of brain
-algia, odynia	pain
-glia	neuroglia
-paresis	incomplete paralysis
-plegia	paralysis

2. Anatomical terms

(1) Nerve

axon
dentrite
ganglion
myelin sheath
nerve cell, ganglion cell
nerve ending
neurofibril
neuroglia
neuron
Nissl's body
synapse

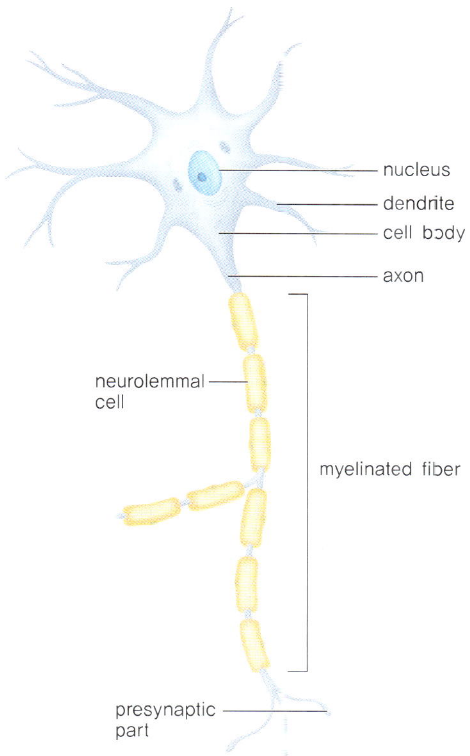

그림 7-7. Parts of a neuron and the pathway of a nervous impulse

(2) Nervous system

arachnoid	midbrain
brain stem	pachymeninges, dura mater
cerebellumparasym	pathetic nerve
cerebrospinal fluid	piamater
cerebrum	pons
gray matter	spinal cord
leptomeninges	sympathetic nerve
medulla oblongatawhite matter	

(3) Cranial nerve

Ⅰ. olfactory nerve	Ⅶ. facial nerve
Ⅱ. optic nerve	Ⅷ. vestibulocochlear nerve
Ⅲ. oculomotor nerve	Ⅸ. glossopharyngeal nerve
Ⅳ. trochlear nerve	Ⅹ. vagus nerve
Ⅴ. trigeminal nerve	Ⅺ. accessory nerve
Ⅵ. abducens nerve	Ⅻ. hypoglossal nerve

(4) Spinal nerve

cervical nerves	sacral nerves
thoracic nerves	coccygeal nerves
lumbar nerves	

(5) Classification of brain

diemcephalon	hypothalamus
	thalamencephalon
mesencephalo	pedun culus cerebri
	tectum mesencephali
mesencephalo	cerbellum
	pons
myelencephalon	medulla oblongata
telencephalon	corpus striatum
	hemispherium
	rhinencephalon

3. Medical terms

Alzheimer's disease : dementia of unknown etiology begining at middle age.

anencephaly : congenital abscence of the cranial vault, with the cerebral hemispheres completely missing or reduced small masses.

aphasia : defect or loss of the power of expression by speech, writing, or signs, or of comprehension of spoken or written language, due to disease or injury of the brain centers.

ataxia : failure of muscular coordination ; irregularity of muscular action.

Bells palsy : neuropathy of the facial nerve, resulting in paralysis of the muscles of the face, usually on one side.

brain death : irreversible brain damage as manifested by absolute unresponsiveness to all stimuli, absence of all muscle activity, including respiration.

cerebral angiography : radiography of the vascular system of the brain after injection of contrast materia into the artery.

cerebral concussion : loss of consciousness, transient or prolonged, due to a blow to the head.

cerebral contusion : injury to tissues without breakage of skin ; a bruise.

cerebral embolism : an embolus is a small mass of material circulating in the blood vessel. It can consist of air, fat, or other material introduced into the circulatory system.

cerebral meningitis : inflammation of the meninges of the brain.

cerebral palsy : a persisting qualitative motor disorder appearing before the age of three years, due to a nonprogressive damage to the brain.

cerebral thrombosis : a thrombus, or clot, in a blood vessel of the brain is by far the most common cause of stroke.

chordotomy : surgical division of the anterolateral tracts of the spinal cord.

coma : a state of unconsciousness from which the patient cannot be aroused, even by powerful stimuli. Harvard Medical school to examine the definition of brain death established criteria for determining irreversible coma or brain death.

convulsion : a series of involuntary contractions of the voluntary muscles. Convulsions can be produced by hypoglycemia, hypocalcemia, brain cell injury (head trauma, tumors), anoxia, cerebral hemorrhage and edema, infection and high fever.

craniotomy : any operation on the cranium.

decompression : relief of pressure on the intracraniumor the spinal cord by means of surgery.

dementia : permanent loss of mental function.

diplegia : paralysis of like parts on either side of the body.

encephalitis : inflammation of the brain.

encephalography : roentgenography demonstration the intracranial fluid-containing spaces after the withdrawal of cerebrospinal fluid and introduction of air or other gas; it includes pneumoencephalography and ventriculography.

encephalomyelitis : inflammation involving both the brain and the spinal cord.

endarterectomy : excision of the thickened, atheromatous tunica intima of an atery.

epilepsy : paroxysmal transient disturbances of brain function that may be manifested as episodic impairement or loss of comsciousness.

ganglionectomy : excision of a ganglion.

glioma : a tumor composed of neuroglia in any of its states of development.

hematoma : a localized collection of extravasated blood usually clotted, in an organ.

hemiplegia : paralysis of one side of the body : usually caused by a brain lesion, such as a tumor, or by a cerebral vascular accident.

Huntingtons chorea : a rare hereditary disease characterized by quick involuntary movements, speech disturbances and mental deterioration to degenerative changes in the cerebral cortex and basal ganglia.

hydrocephalus : a condition characterized by enlargement of the cranium caused by abnormal accumulation of cerebrospinal fluid within the cerebral ventricular system.

hyperesthesia : a state of abnormally increased sensitivity to stimuli.

hyperventilation : a state in which there is an increased amount of air entering the pumonary alveoli.

hypothermia : a low body temperature.

lethargy : a condition of drowsiness or indifference.

meningioma : a hard, usually vascular tumor occurring mainly along the meningeal vessels and superior longitudinal sinus invading the dura and skull.

meningitis : inflammation of the meninges.

meningocele : hernial protrusion of meninges through a defect in the skull or vertebral column.

multiple sclerosis : demyelination of the white matter of the brain and spinal cord occurring in scattered patches, and resulting in a chronic disabling condition characterized by visual disturbances, weakness, tremors and paralysis.

myasthenia gravis : muscular debility or weakness.

myelitis : inflammation of the spinal cord.

myelography : radiography of the spinal cord after injection of contrast material into the subarachnoid space.

neuralgia : pain in a nerve or along the course of one or more nerves.

neurectomy : the excision of a part of a nerve.

neuritis : inflammation of a nerve; also used to denote noninflammatory lesions of the peripheral nervous system.

neuroma : a tumor or new growth largely made up of nerve cells and nerve fibers.

neuromyelitis : inflammation of nervous and medullary substance.

nystagmus : involuntary, rapid, rhythmic movement(horizontal, vertical, rotatory or mixed).

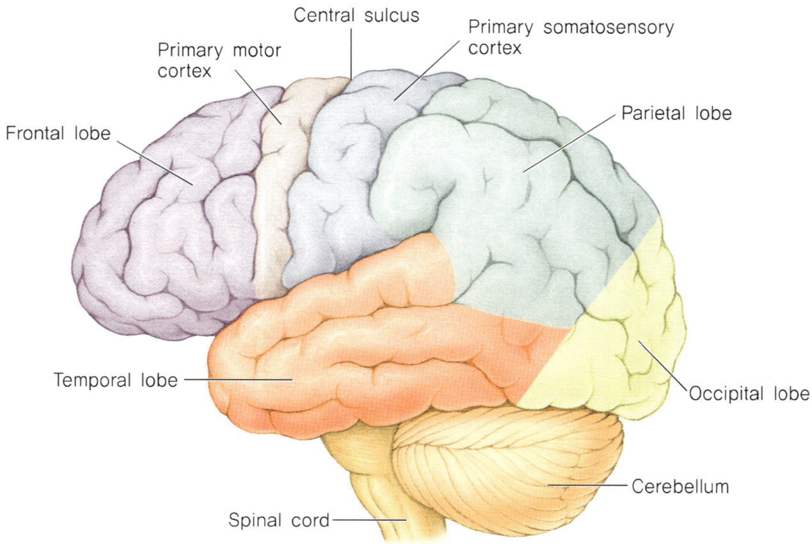

그림 7-8. Functional areas of the cerebrum

paralysis agitans : called also Parkinson's disease and shaking palsy.

paraplegia : paralysis of the legs and, in some cases, the lower part of the body.

Parkinson's disease : a slowly progressive disease usually occuring in later life, characterized pathologically by degeneration within the nuclear masses of the extrapyramidal system, and clinically by masklike faces, tremor of resting muscle, a slowing of voluntary movements, a festinating gait, muscular weakness.

poliomyelitis : an acute, contagious viral disease that attacks the central nervous system, injuring or destroying the nerve cells that control the muscles and sometimes causing paralysis ; called also polio and infantile paralysis.

polioencephalitis : inflammatory disease of the gray matter of the brain.

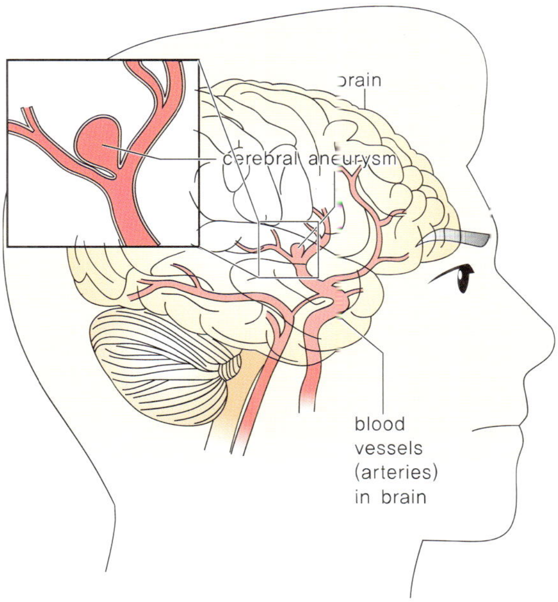

그림 7-9. Ventriculography

polyneuritis : inflammation of many nerves simultaneously.

pyencephalus : intracerebral encapsulated collection of pus.

sciatica : neuralgia along the course of the sciatic nerve.

spina bifida : a developmental anomaly characterized by defective closure of the bony encasement of the spinal cord through which the spinal cord and meninges may or may not protrude.

syncope : a temporary suspension of consciousness due to cerebral anemia ; fainting.

tetraplegia : paralysis of all four extremities ; quadriplegia.

tremor : an involuntary trembling of the body or limbs. It may have either a physical or a psychologic cause.

trigeminal neuralgia : pain arising from irritation of the fifth cranial (trigeminal) nerve. Called also tic douloureux.

ventriculography : radiography of the head after injection of contrast material into the cerebral ventricles.

Chapter 8

PSYCHONEURAL SYSTEM

I. Function of the system

1. Word root

anthrop/o	man, human
gnos/o	knowledge
hyster/o	hysteria
narc/o	stupor
neur/o	nerve
physi/o	physiology, nature
psych/o, ment/o, phren-	mind
schiz/o	division
somat/o, corpor-	body
somn/o, hypn/o	sleep
-mnesia	remember
-philia	abnormal fondness
-phobia	abnormal fear
-phoria	abnoral feeling
-somnia	sleep
-thymia	ondition of mind

2. Medical terms

acrophobia : morbid dread of high places.

affective psychosis : the various forms of manic depressive psychosis, characterized by a severe disorder of mood.

agoraphobia : fear of being in a large open space.

alcoholism : the extreme dependence on excessive amounts of alcohol, associated with a cumulative pattern of deviant behaviors.

amentia : congenital mental retardation of varying extent.

amnesia : pathologic impairment of memory.

anxiety : a feeling of uncertainty and fear without apparent stimulus.

aphasia : defect or loss of the power of expression by speech, writing, or signs, or of comprehension of spoken or written language, due to disease or injury of the brain centers.

auditory halluciation : the hearing of unreal sounds.

aura : a peculiar sensation preceding the appearance of more definite symptoms. An epileptic aura precedes the convulsive seizure and may involve visual diturbances, dizziness, numbness, or any of a number of sensation which the patient may find difficult to describe exactly.

autism : a form of thinking in which the content is either entirely subjective or has a subjective meaning and emphasis including fantasies, delusions, and hallucinations; a fundamental symptom of schizophrenia.

automatism, automatic behavior : the performance of nonreflex acts without conscious volition.

behavioral therapy : a therapeutic approach in which the focus is on the patient's observable behavior.

compulsion : an overwhelming urge to perform an irrational act or ritual.

delirium : a mental disturbances of relatively short duration usually reflecting a toxic state, marked by illusions, hallucinations, delusions, excitement, restlessness, and incoherence.

delusion : a false personal belief based on incorrect inference about extenal reality and firmly maintained in spite of incontrovertible and obvious proof or evidence to the contrary.

dementia : organic loss of intellectual function.

depression : a morbid sadness, rejection, or melancholy, distinguished from grief, which is realistic and proportionate to a personal loss.

disorientation : the loss of proper bearings, or a state of mental confusion as to time, place, or identity.

electric shock(convulsive) therapy : a form of shock therapy that is most effective in the treatment of depression.

electroencephalography : the recording of the electric currents developed in the brain.

epilepsy : a group of neurological disorders characterized by recurrent episodes of convulsive seizures, sensory disturbances, abnormal behavior, loss of consciousness, or all of these. Common to all types of epilesy is an uncontrolled electrical discharge from the nerve cells of the cerebral cortex.

euphoria : bodily comfort. In psychiatry, abnormal or exaggerated sense of well being.

exhibitionism : when severe leads to exposure of the genitals, sometimes accompanied by sexual gratification.

family therapy : group therapy in which the patient and his family are treated together.

fetishism : the adoration of an inanimate object as a symbol of a loved person.

fever therapy : treatment of disease by induction of high body temperature.

focal seizure : a transitory disturbance in motor, sensory, or autonomic function resulting from abnormal neuronal discharges in a localized part of the brain, most frequently motor or sensory areas adjacent to the fissure of Rolando. Also called Jacksonian seizure.

grand mal seizure : an epileptic seizure characterized by a generalized involuntary muscular contraction and cessation of respiration followed by tonic and clonic spasms of the muscles.

grandiose delusions : delusional conviction of one's own importance, power, wealth, ect.

group psychotherapy : psychotherapy carried out with a group of patients or the relatives of patients or both.

hallucination : a sensory impression(sight, touch, sound, smell, or taste) that has no basis in external stimulation.

hypnotherapy : the use of hypnosis in the treatment of disease.

hypochondriasis : abnormal concern about ones health.

illusion : a mental impression derived from misinterpretation of an acute sensory stimulation.

insomnia : inability to sleep.

insulin shock treatment : a form of shock therapy employed in the treatment of schizophrenia.

involutional melanchloia : a major depression occurring in late middle life.

Korsakoff's syndrome : psychosis associated with chronic alcoholism and caused by vitamin B_1 deficiency; characteristics include disturbances of orientation, memory defect, susceptibility to external stimulation and suggestion, hallucinations, and, usually, the signs of polyneuritis.

mannerism : a stereotyped movement or habit.

mania : a disordered mental state of extreme excitement; specifically, the manic type of manic depressive psychosis.

melancholia : a mental state characterized by extreme sadness or depression, with inhibition of mental and physical activity.

milieu therapy : daily participation in group psychiatric therapy at a hospital.

narci(ssi)sm : self love, which may or may not include genital excitation.

narcolepsy : a condition marked by an uncontrollable desire for sleep.

nightmare : a terrifying dream.

obsession : an unwanted idea or impulse that repeatedly intrudes into consciousness. Morbid obsession may dominate the mind and lead to irrational actions that are an attempt to escape the obsessional thoughts.

pedophilia : sexual activity of adults with children as the objects.

persecutory delusions : a morbid belief on the part of a patient that he is being injuried by secret enemies.

petit mal seizure : an epileptic seizure characterized by a sudden, momentary loss of consciousness occasionally accompanied by minor myoclonus of the neck or upper extremities, slight symmetrical twitching of the face, or a loss of muscle tone. The seizures usually occur many times a day without a warning aura and are most frequent in children and adolescents, especially at the time of puberty.

phobia : any persistent abnormal dread or fear that appears to result from repressed inner conflicts of which the affected person is not aware.

psychoanalysis : method of eliciting from patients an idea of their past emotional experiences.

psychological test : any test to measure one's development, personality, intelligence, thought, etc.

sexual sadism : sexual perversion in which satisfaction is derived from hurting another.

social therapy : any treatment emphasizing socioenvironmental and interpersonal rather than intrapsychic factors.

somnambulism : habitual walking in the sleep.

thematic apperception test : a projective test in which the subject tells a story based on each of a pictures.

transsexualism : desire to change one's anatomic sex.

Chapter 9 CARDIOVASCULAR SYSTEM

Heart Lies in the mediastinum(between the lungs). Has four chambers : right and left atria(singular, atrium) are receiving chambers (also called auricle) ; right and left ventricles are pumping chambers. The apex is the pointed part(bottom of the heart). The function of the heart is to pump blood, thereby maintaining circulation.

Valves : keep blood from backflowing.

tricuspid : between right atrium and right ventricle.

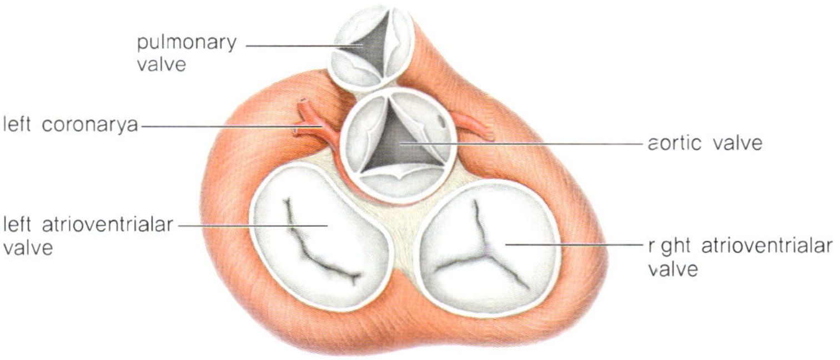

그림 9-1. Cross section of heart showing coronary arteries. Also showing anatomic relationship of right ventricle, RV, to left ventricle, LV and globular shape of left ventricle and half-moon shape of right ventricle as it drapes around left ventricle. RA as right auricle; LA, left auricle.

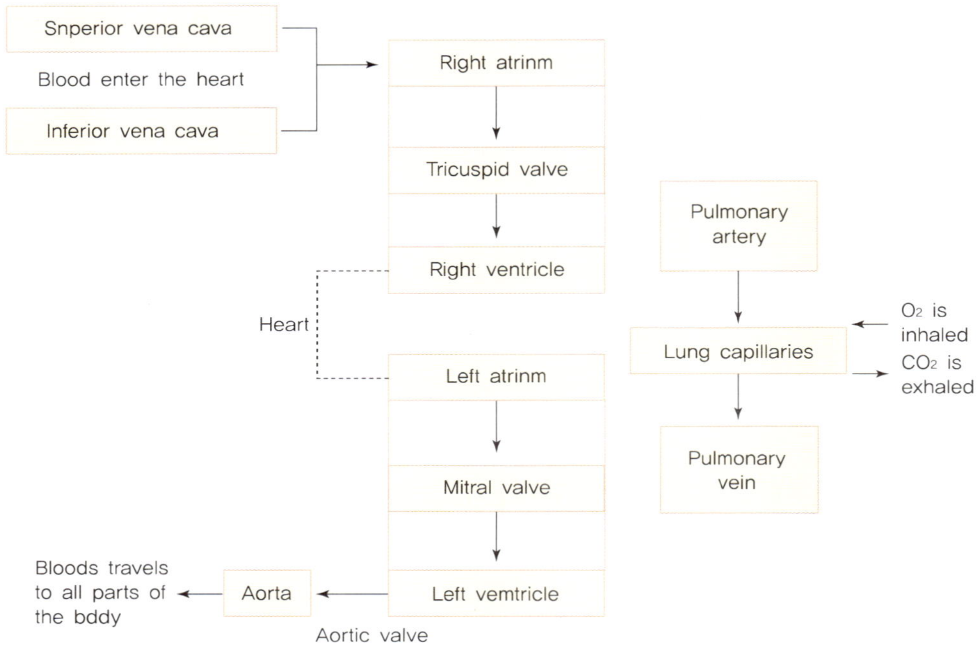

그림 9-2. Pathway of blood through the heart

Pulmonary semilunar : between right ventricle and pulmonary artery.

mitral : between left atrium and left ventricle(also called bicuspid valve).

aortic : between left ventricle and aorta.

septum : divides the right and left sides of the heart.

muscle : myocardium is the heart muscle.

membranes : endocardium lines inside of heart chambers ; pericardium is the outer double membranous sac ; epicardium(visceral layer) ; and outer parietal layer.

Conduction system

sinoatrial node or SA node : this is the pacemaker(right atrium).

atrioventricular node : in septum.

bundle of His : conducting fibers.

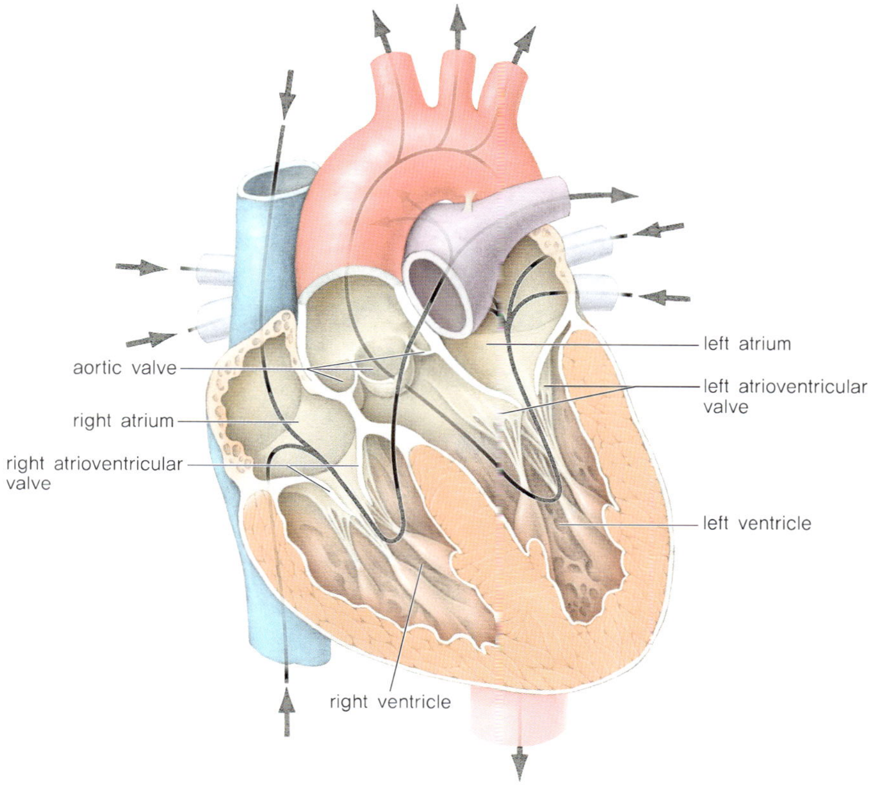

그림 9-3. Circulation in the normal heart. The right side of the heart sends the blood to the lungs(pulmonary circulation) ; the left side sends blood to the entire body(systemic circulation). Light areas contain oxygenated blood.

circulation The function of circulation is to carry oxygen and nutrients to cells and to carry carbon dioxide and wastes away from the cells.

pulmonary circulation : right side of heart-blood returning from the body is received in the right atrium, goes to right ventricle and through the pulmonary artery to the lungs. It returns to the left atrium by way of the pulmonary veins.

systemic circulation : from left atrium, blood flows to the left ventricle and is pumped out through the aortic valve to the aorta and goes to the entire body.

portal circulation : circulation from the intestines, stomach, pancreas and spleen to the liver.

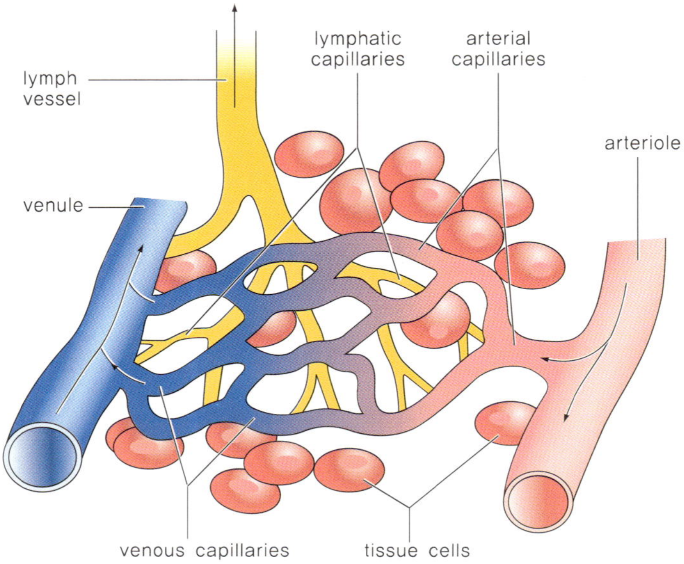

그림 9-4. Capillary bed showing lymphatic vessels and how tiny arterioles connect with tiny venules. The gaseous and nutrient exchanges take place in these capillary beds.

Blood vessels : arteries, veins, capillaries.

arteries : always carry blood away from the heart(oxygenated blood except in pulmonary arteries).

veins : always carry blood toward the heart(deoxygenated blood except in pulmonary veins).

aorta : largest artery(ascending, aortic arch, thoracic, and abdominal sections).

vena cava : largest vein(superior and inferior venae cavae).

coronary arteries : supply the heart muscle with blood(arise from the base of the aorta). Occlusion of these causes heart attack (coronary occlusion).

I. Heart

1. Word root

angi/o, vas/o	vessel
aort/o	aorta
arteri/o	artery
atri/o	atrium
cardi/o, coron/o	heart
cyan/o	blue
phleb/o, ven/o	vein
valv/o	valve
ventricul/o	ventricle

2. Anatomical terms

atrioventricular node(A-V node)	pulmonic valve
chorda tendineae	semilunar valve
coronary artery	sino-atrial node(S-A node)
diastole	systole
foramen ovale	tricuspid valve
mitral valve, bicuspid valve	

3. Medical terms

abdominal aortography : roentgenogrphy of arteries after injection of contrast material into the abdomanal aorta.

Adams-Stokes disease : a condition caused by heart block and characterized by sudden attacks of unconsciousness with or without convulsions ; called also syncope.

angina pectoris : a paroxysmal thoracic pain caused most often by myocardial anoxia owing to atherosclerosis of the coronary arteries.

angiocardiography : roentgenography of the heart and great vessels after introduction of contrast material into a blood vessel.

angioplasty : surgical repair of blood vessels or lymphatic channels.

aortic stenosis : a narrowing of the aortic orifice of the heart or of the aorta itself.

arrythmia : any variation from the normal rhythm of the heartbeat, including sinus arrythmia, premature beat, heart block, atrial fibrillation, atrial flutter.

artificial cardiac pacemaker : a device designed to stimulate, by electrical impulses, contraction of the heart muscle at a certain rate.

artificial respiration : maintained by artificial means.

atrial fibrillation : atrial arrythmia characterized by rapid randomized contractions of the atrial myocardium, causing totally irregular, often rapid ventricular rate.

atrial flutter : a condition of cardiac arrythmia in which the atrial contractions are rapid (200 to 320 per minute), but regular.

atrial septal defect : a congenital heart defect in which there is persistent patency of the atrial septum, owing to failure of closure of the ostium primum or ostium secundum.

Blalock-Taussig operation : the anastomosis of the subclavian artery to the pulmonary artery in order to shunt some of the systemic circulation into the pulmonary circulation.

bradycardia : slowness of the heart rate, as evidenced by slowing of the pulse rate to less than 60.

cardiac catheterization : the insertion of a catheter into a vein or artery and guiding it into the interior of the heart for purposes of measuring cardiac output, determining the oxygen content of blood in the heart chambers, and evaluating the structual components of the heart.

cardiac massage : repeated, rhythmic compression of the heart applied directly, during surgery, or through the intact chest wall in an effort to maintain circulation after cardiac arrest or ventricular fibrillation.

cardiac pacing : regulation of the rate of contraction of the heart muscle by an artificial cardiac pacemaker.

cardiocentesis : surgical puncture into the pericardial space and aspiration of fluid for therapeutic or diagnostic purposes.

cardiomegaly : cardiac hypertrophy

cardiopulmonary resuscitation : the reestablishing of heart and lung action as indicated for cardiac arrest.

coarctation of aorta : a localized malformation characterized by deformity of the tunica media of the aorta, causing narrowing, usually severe, of the lumen of the vessel.

congestive heart failure : heart disease characterized by breathlessness and abnormal sodium and water retention, resulting in edema.

coronary ateriography : roentgenography of arteries after injection of contrast material into the coronary artery

cyanosis : a bluish discoloration, applied especially to such discoloration of skin, mucous membranes due to excessive concentration of reduced hemoglobin in the blood.

dextroposition of aorta : displacement to the right of the aorta.

echocardiography : a method of graphically recording the position and motion of the heart wall or internal structures by the ultrasonic waves.

electrocardiography : the graphic recording from the body surface of the potential of electric currents generated by the heart, as means of studying the action of the heart muscle.

endocarditis : an abnormal condition that affects the endocardium and the heart valves. The kinds of endocarditis are bacterial endocarditis, nonbacterial endocarditis.

extracorporeal circulation : the circulation of blood outside the body as through a hemodialyzer for removal of substances usually excreted in the urine, or through a heart-lung machine for carbon dioxide-oxygen exchange.

hypothermia therapy : the reduction of a patients body temperature to counteract high prolonged fever caused by an infectious or neurologic disease, or, less frequently, as an adjunct to anesthesia in heart or brain surgery.

insufficiency : inability to perform a necessary adequately. Some kinds of insufficiency are mitral insufficiency, aortic insufficiency.

murmur : an auscultatory sound, benign or pathologic, particularly a periodic sound of short duration of cardiac or vascular origin.

myocardial infarction : an occlusion of a coronary artery, caused by atherosclerosis or an embolus that results in a necrotic area in the vasculature myocardium.

myocarditis : inflammation of the muscle walls of the heart.

open heart surgery : surgery that involves incision into one or more chambers of the hearts.

palpitation : sensation of an unduly rapid or irregular heart beat.

pancarditis : an abnormal condition characterized by inflammation of the entire heart, including the endocardium, myocardium, and pericardium.

patent ductus arteriosus : abnormal persistance of an open lumen in the ductus arteriosus, between the aorta and the pulmonary artery, after birth.

patent foramen ovale : the septal opening in the fetal heart that provides a communication between the atria. The opening closes at birth; failure to close results in atrial septal defect.

pentalogy of Gasul : the four defects included in the tetralogy of Fallot, occurring in association with patent foramen ovale or atrial septal defect.

pericardial effusion : the escape of fluid into a cavity of pericardium.

pericardial punture : surgical punture into the pericardial spaces.

pericardiectomy : excision of pericardium.

pericarditis : an inflammation of the pericardium owing to trauma, malignant neoplastic disease, infection, uremia, myocardial infarction, collagen disease, or idiopathic causes.

precordialgia : pain in the precordium.

pulmonary stenosis : narrowing of the opening between the pulmonary artery and the right ventricle.

regurgitation : a backward flowing, as the casting up of undigested food or the backward flowing of blood into the heart, or between the chambers of the heart when a valve is incompetent.

rheumatic heart disease : heart disease caused by rheumatic fever, consisting chiefly of valvular deformities.

stenosis : narrowing or structure of a duct or canal.

sternotomy : incision of the sternum.

tachycardia : excessive rapidity in the action of the heart; the term is usually applied to a heart rate above 100 per minute.

tetralogy of Fallot : a combination of congenital cardiac defects, namely, pulmonary stenosis, ventricular septal defects, dextroposition of the aorta, so that it overides the interventricular septum and receives venous as well as arterial blood, and right ventricular hypertrophy.

valvulotomy : incision of a valve such as a valve of the heart; called also valvotomy.

ventricular septal defect : a congenital heart defect in which there is persistent patency of the ventricular septum on either the muscular or fibrous portion most often due to failure of the bulbar septum to completely close the interventricular foramen. The defect permits flow of blood directly from one ventricle to the other, resulting in bypassing of the pulmonary circulation and producing varying degrees of cyanosis because of oxygen deficiency.

Ⅱ. Vascular system

1. Word root

aneurysm/o	aneurysm
angi/o, vas/o	vessel
arteri/o	artery
arteriol/o	small artery
hemangi/o	blood vessel
ox/o	oxygen
phleb/o, ven/o	vein
sphygm/o	pulse
steth/o	chest
valv/o, valvul/o	valve
varic/o	swollen vein
venul/o	small vein

2. Anatomical terms

aorta	right lymphatic duct
arteriole	sinusoid
artery	spleen
capillary	systemic circulation
greater circulation	thoracic duct
hilus lienis	tunica externa
lesser circulation	tunica intima
lymph node	tunica media
portal vein	vein
pulmonary circulation	vena cava
reticuloendothelial cell	venule

3. Medical terms

acrocyanosis : cyanosis of extremities.

aneurysm : a sac formed by the localized dilatation of the wall of an artery, vein, or the heart.

aneurysmectomy : excision of an aneurysm.

angiospasm : spastic contraction of the blood vessels; called also vasospasm.

angiostomy : the operation of making an opening into a blood vessel.

arteriolitis : inflammation of the arterioles.

arteriosclerosis : a group of diseases characterized by thickening and loss of elasticity of the arterial walls, popularly called hardening of the arteries.

arteritis : inflammation of artery.

atherosclerosis : an extremely common form of arteriosclerosis in which deposits of yellowing plaques(atheromas) containing cholesterol, other lipoid material.

bubo : an enlarged and inflamed lymph node, particularly in the axilia or groin, due to such infections as plague, syphilis, gonorrhea, lymphogranuloma venereum, and tuberculosis.

embolectomy : surgical removal of an embolus.

embolism : the sudden blocking of an artery by a clot of foreign material(embolus) that has been brought to its site of lodgment by blood current.

endarterectomy : excision of thickened atheromatous areas of the innermost coat of an artery.

endarteritis : inflammation of the innermost coat(tunica intima) of an artery.

Hodgkins disease : a malignant condition characterized by painless, progressive enlargement of the lymph nodes, spleen and general lymphoid tissue; other symptoms may include anorexia, lassitude, weight loss, fever, pruritus, night sweats, and anemia.

Homan's sign : discomfort behind the knee on forced dorsiflexion of the foot ; a sign of thrombosis in the veins of the calf.

hypertension : persistently high blood pressure. In adults, it is generally agreed that a blood pressure is abnormally high when the systolic is equal to or greater than 140 mmHg and the diastolic pressure is equal to or greater than 90 mmHg.

infarction : formation of necrosed tissue due to the occlusion or stenosis of supplying artery.

Leriche's syndrome : a syndrome caused by obstruction of the terminal aorta, usally occuring in males.

lymphosarcoma : a general term applied to malignant neoplastic disorders of lymphoid tissue, but not including Hodgkins disease.

Pel-Ebstein's fever : a cyclic fever occasionally seen in Hodgkins disease and also associated with other diseases, characterized by irregular episodes of pyrexia of several days duration, with intervening afebrile periods lasting for days or weeks. Called also Pel-Ebstein pyrexia, and Pel-Ebstein symptoms.

periarteritis : inflammation of the externa coats of an artery and of the tissue around the artery.

phlebectasia : dilatation of a vein; called also varicosity.

phlebitis : inflammation of vein.

phleborrhaphy : suture of a vein.

phlebosclerosis : fibrous thickening of the walls of veins.

phlebotomy : incision of a vein.

polyarteritis : a condition marked by multiple sites of inflammatory and destructive lesions in the arterial system.

Raynaud's phenmenon : spasm of arterioles, usally in the digits(and nose or ear), with intermittent pallor or cyanosis of the skin.

splenectomy : excision of spleen.

sympathectomy : the transection, resection of some portion of the sympathetic nervous pathways.

thrombectomy : surgical removal of a clot from a blood vessel.

thromboangitis : inflammation of a blood vessel, with thrombosis.

thromboangitis obliterans : thromboangitis with contraction of the vessel about the clot leading to diminution of blood flow distal to the site; most frequently the lower extremities are affected called also Buergers disease.

thrombophlebitis : inflammation of a vein associated with thrombus formation.

thrombosis : formation, development, or presence of a thrombus.

varicose veins : swollen, distended, and knotted veins, usually in the subcutaneous tissues of the leg. They result from a stagnated or sluggish blow of the blood, in combination with defective valves and weakened walls of the veins.

vasoconstriction : the diminution of the caliber of vessels, especially constriction of arterioles leading to decreased blood flow to a part.

vasodilatation : a state of increased caliber of the blood vessels.

veinstripping : excision of lengths of large veins and the use of a stripper.

venesection : phlebotomy.

venipuncture : surgical puncture of a vein.

Chapter

10 BLOOD AND LYMPHATIC SYSTEM

Ⅰ. Blood

red blood cells(RBCs) : are called erythrocytes ; they contain hemoglobin, which carries oxygen to the cells and carries carbon dioxide away from the cells.

white blood cells(WBCs) : are called leukocytes. There are five basic kinds of white blood cells.

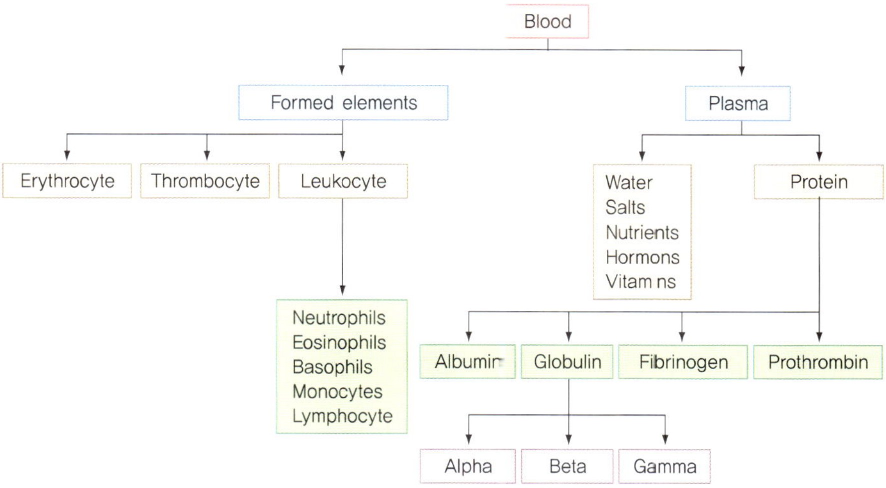

그림 10-1. Composition of blood

A. Granulocytes(have granules in cytoplasm) are formed in bone marrow. There are three types :

1. Neutrophils : also called polymorphonuclear leukocytes or PMNs because their nuclei have many shapes or forms. They defend the body by means of phagocytosis(ingesting invaders).
2. Eosinophils : are thought to be active and increased in parasites infection.
3. Basophils : increased in allergy reaction.

B. Agranulocytes(have no granules in cytoplasm) are produced by spleen and lymph nodes. There are two types :

4. Lymphocytes : produce antibodies and destroy foreign material.
5. Monocytes : perform phagocytosis and destruction of invaders.

plasma : is the liquid part of the blood, minus the cells. It is amber colored. If whole blood is allowed to stand in a container, the cells will settle to the bottom(clot), and the clear plasma will rise to the top.

serum : is plasma minus the fibrinogen that promotes clotting.

platelets : are also called thrombocytes(clotting particles).

reticulocyte : immature red blood cell, in bone marrow.

Blood types

Landsteiner types : based on type of red blood cells : A, B, AB, and O. (Type O is sometimes referred to as a universal donor ; and type AB is sometimes referred to as a universal recipient.)

distribution : our population shows 3% AB, 10% B, 40% to 44% A, and 40% to 44% O. When incompatible bloods are mixed, clumping of cells occurs. Example : Type A red cells that are dropped into type B blood cause clumping or sticking together.

These clumps could cause fatal injury as they pass through the heart or brain.

type and crossmatch(x-match) : before a transfusion is given, this is done to determine compatibility. Cells from the donor and serum from the recipient are mixed to see if clumping occurs. A second test may also done using the cells of the recipient and the serum of the donor. If no clumping occurs, it can be assumed that the two bloods are of the same type.

Because of possible complications resulting from even the most carefully handled transfusion, they are being done less frequently. Individuals who must still receive transfused blood, and who are able to prepare for their operations, may bank their own blood in advance.

Rh Factor so named because it was first found in the blood of the Rhesus monkey.

85% of population have this factor, called Rh+.

15% do not have this factor ; they are Rh-.

The Rh factor acts like a foreign substance to anyone who is negative. If an Rh-negative person received Rh-positive blood, that persons own blood will make a substance called an antibody, which will act against the Rh-positive blood. If an Rh-negative woman mates with an Rh-positive man, their child may inherit the Rh factor from his father. The mothers blood may produce so many antibodies against it that the baby may die before or shortly after birth. This does not usually affect the first child of these parents because not enough antibodies are present, but will affect subsequent pregnancies.

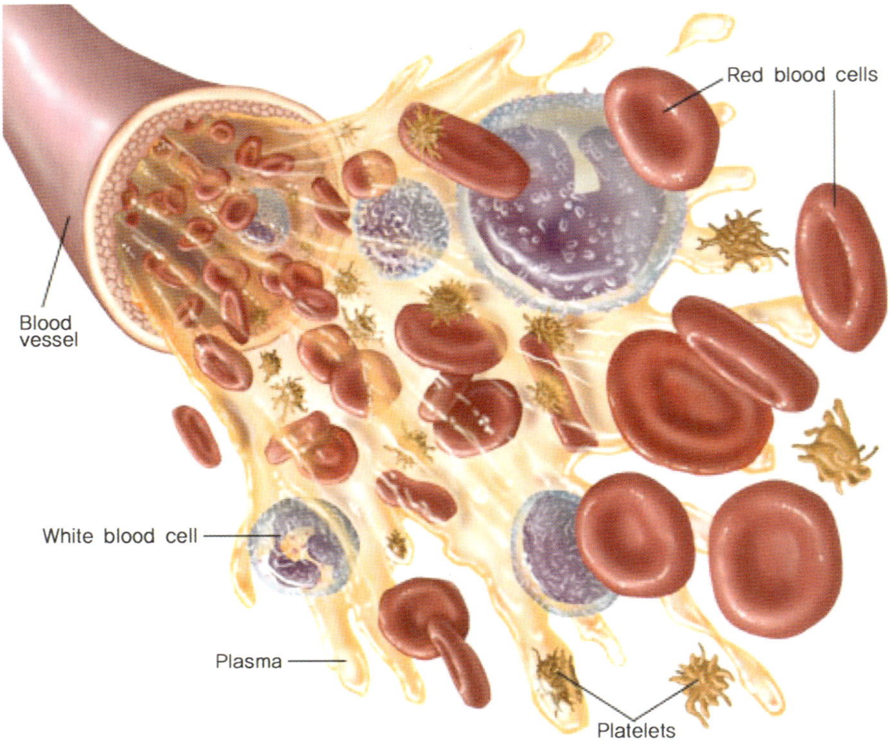

그림 10-2. Types of blood cells

Antibody titers(tests) done during pregnancy aid the doctor in determining when intervention is necessary.

If the titer rises rapidly, the pregnancy can be terminated early or preparation for exchange transfusion at time of delivery can be made.

RhoGAM can be given to the Rh-negative mother following her first delivery. This prevents Rh antibodies from forming.

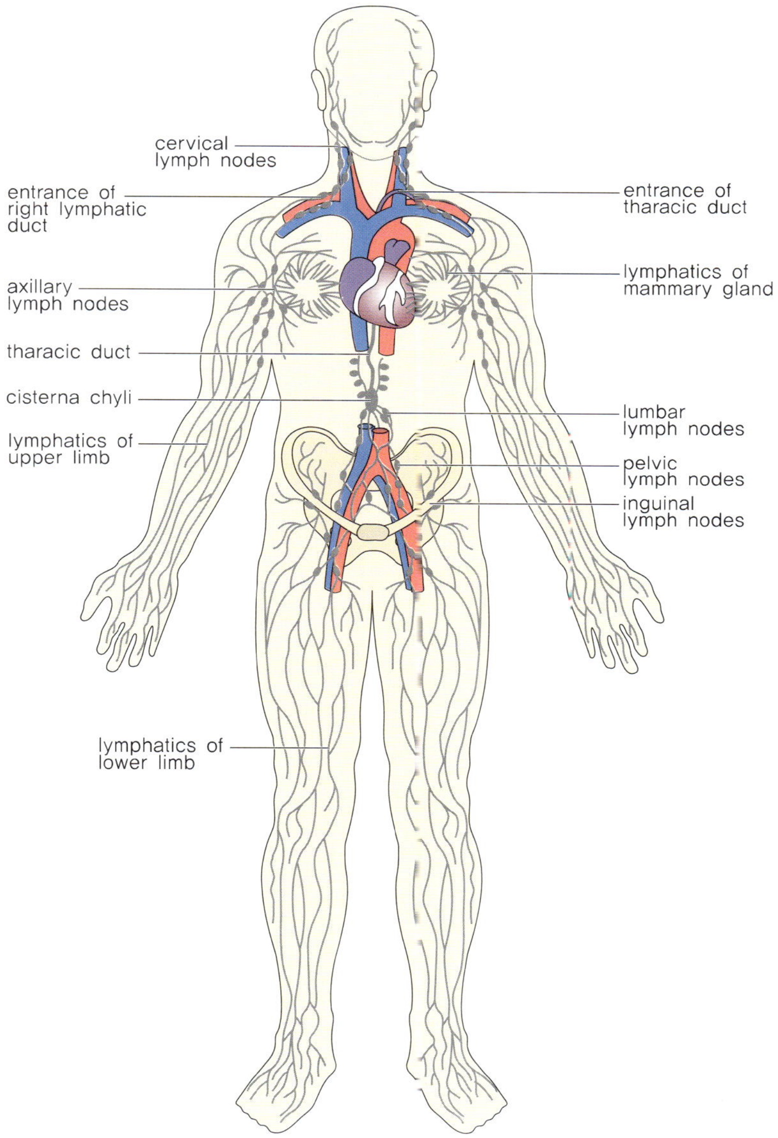

그림 10-3. Lymphatic system

Ⅱ. Lymphatic vessels, lymph nodes, spleen

Lymph fluid comes from the blood ; it filters out into the spaces between tissue cells, and returns to the blood via lymphatic vessels. Lymph nodes are numerous in certain parts of the body ; nodes are palpable in the neck(cervical nodes), in the axilla(axillary nodes), and in the groin(inguinal nodes) ; they help filter out harmful substances such as bacteria and cancer cells. The spleen is the largest lymphatic organ of the body. In youth it helps build up blood cells ; it also destroys old blood cells.

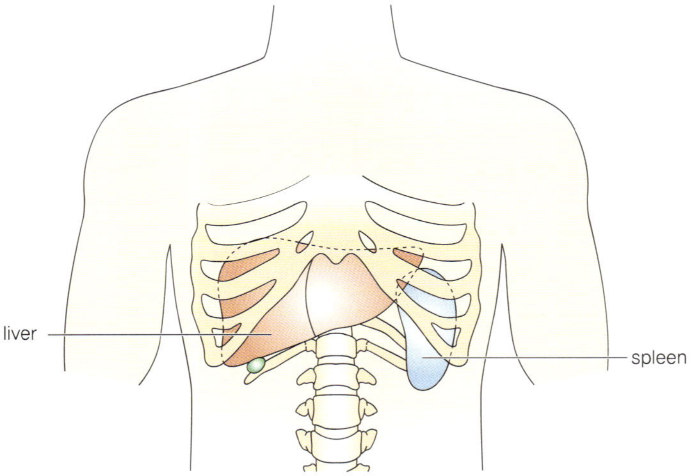

그림 10-4. The spleen and adjacent organs

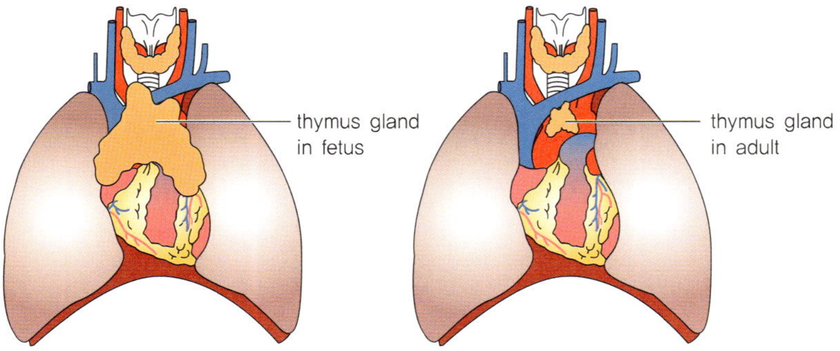

그림 10-5. The thymus gland

Ⅲ. Function of the system

1. Word root

aden/o	gland
anis/o	unequal
blast/o	germ, immature cell
cyt/o	cell
erythr/o	red
granul/o	granules
hem/o, hemat/o	blood
hist/o, histi/o	tissue
is/o	same, equal
leuk/o	white
lymph/o	lymph
lymphangi/o	lymph vessel
myel/o	bone marrow
phag/o	eat, swallow
reticul/o	network
splen/o, lien/o	spleen
thromb/o	clot
thym/o	thymus gland
-emia	blood condition
-osis	abnormal increase
-penia	abnormal reduction
-poiesis	formation

2. Anatomical terms

agranulocyte	leukocyte
basophil	lymphocyte
eosinophil	monocyte
erythrocyte	neutrophil
fibrin	plasma
fibrinogen	platelet
granulocyte	prothrombin
hemoglobin	serum

3. Medical terms

agranulocytosis : an acute disease in which there is a sudden drop in the production of leukocytes, leaving the body defenseless against bacterial invasion. Laboratory tests reveal a profound leukopenia.

anemia : a reduction below normal in the number of erythrocyte.

anisocytosis : the presence in the blood of erythrocytes showing abnormal variation in size.

aplastic anemia : a form of anemia generally unresponsive to specific antianemia therapy, often accompanied by granulocytopenia and thrombocytopenia, in which the bone marrow may not necessarily be acellular or hypoplastic but fails to produce adequate numbers of blood elements.

basophilia : basophilic leukocytosis.

blood transfusion : the introduction of whole blood or blood component directly into the blood stream.

Burkitt's lymphoma : a highly undifferentiated B cell lymphoma.

dyscrasia : a morbid condition, usually referring to an imbalance of component elements.

enlarged lymph nodes : increase in volume of lymph nodes.

eosionophilia : the formation and accumulation of an abnormally large number of eosinophils in the blood.

erythrocytosis : increase in the total red cell mass secondary to any of a number of nonhematogenic systemic disorders in response to a known stimulus(secondary polycythemia), in contrast to primary polycythemia (polycythemia vera).

erythropenia : deficiency in the number of erythrocytes.

folic acid deficiency anemia : anemia characterized by deficiency of folic acid. Folic acid deficiency may result from the inability of the blood to utilize the vitamin.

G6PD deficiency anemia : anemia characterized by deficiency of glucose -6-phosphate(an intermediate in carbohydrate metabolism).

hemochromatosis : a disorder of iron metabolism with excess deposition of iron in the tissues, bronze skin pigmentation, cirrhosis of the liver, and diabetes mellitus.

hemophilia : a condition characterized by impaired coagulation of the blood, and a strong tendency to bleed.

hemostasis : the arrest of bleeding by surgical means.

hereditary spherocytic anemia : form of hemolytic anemia characterized by spherocytosis.

hypertrophy of lymphatic gland : enlargement of lymph gland.

infectious mononucleosis : an acute infectious disease that causes changes in the leukocytes; called also glandular fever.

iron deficiency anemia : a form characterized by low or absent iron stores, low serum iron concentration, low hemoglobin concentration or hematocrit, and hypochromic, microcytic red blood corpuscles.

leukemia : a progressive, malignant disease of the blood forming organs, marked by distorted proliferation and development of leukocytes and

their precursors in the blood and bone marrow.
It is accompanied by a reduced number of erythrocytes and blood platelets, resulting in anemia and increased susceptibility to infection and hemorrhage.

leukocytosis : a transient increase in the number of leukocytes in the blood.

leukopenia : reduction of the number of leukocytes in the blood, the count being 5000 or less.

lymphadenectomy : surgical excision of one or more lymph nodes.

lymphadenitis : inflammation of lymph nodes.

lymphadenopathy : disease of the lymph nodes.

lymphadenotomy : incision of a lymph node.

lymphangiectomy : excision of an or more lymphatic vessels.

lymphangiography : roentgenography of the lymphatic vessels following the injection of contrast medium.

lymphangioma : a tumor composed of new formed lymph spaces.

lymphangitis : inflammation of a lymphatic vessles.

lymphedema : accumulation of interstitial fluid as a result of stasis of lymph.

lymphocytic leukemia : leukemia associated with hyperplasia and overactivity of the lymphoid tissue.

lymphocytopenia : an acute or chronic reduction in blood lymphocytes.

lymphocytosis : increase in the number of normal lymphocytes in the blood or in effusion.

macrocytosis : the presence of macrocytes in the blood.

malignant lymphoma : malignant tumor of the lymphoid tissue.

megaloblastic anemia : anemia characterized by the presence of megaloblasts in bone marrow.

megaloblastosis : the presence of a large, nucleated immature progenitor of an abnormal erythrocytic series; megaloblasts are present in the blood in certain anemias.

microcytosis : a condition in which the erythrocytes are smaller than normal.

monocytosis : increase of monocytes in the blood.

neutropenia : diminished number of neutrophils in the blood.

neutrophilia : increase in the number of neutrophils in the blood; it is the most common form of leukocytosis and may result from many causes, among them acute infections, intoxications, hemorrahage, and rapidly growing malignant neoplasms.

non hodgkin's lymphoma : a heterogeneous group of diseases, consisting of neoplastic proliferation of lymphoid cells that usually disseminate throughout the body.

pernicious anemia : a serious anemia that results from lack of secretion by the gastric mucous membrane of a factor(intrinsic factor) essential to formation of erythrocytes and absorption of vitamin B_{12}.

pica : craving for unnatural articles of food; a depraved appetite.

poikilocytosis : the presence of poikilocyte(irregularly shaped red cells in the blood seen in pernicious anemia).

polycythemia : an increase in the total cell mass of the blood. Primary polycythemia(called also polycythemia vera) is a myeloproliferative disorder of unknown ethiology secondary polycythemia is a physiologic condidition resulting from a decreased oxygen supply to the tissues.

purpura : purplish or brownish red discoloration caused by hemorrhage into the tissues.

reticulocytosis : an excess of reticulocytes(a young erythrocyte showing a basophilic reticulum under vital staining) in the peripheral blood.

rouleau(pl. rouleaux) : a roll of red blood cells resembling a pile of coins.

sideroblastic anemia : a form of anemia characterized by a nucleated erythrocyte containing iron granules in its cytoplasm.

sickle cell anemia : a genetically determined defect of hemoglobin synthesis associated with poor physical development and skeletal anomalies, occurring usually in blacks.

spherocyte : a small, globular completely hemoglobinated erythrocyte without the usual central pallor ; characteristically found in hereditary spherocytosis but also in acquired hemolytic anemia.

spherocytosis : the presence of spherocytes in the blood.

thrombocytopenia : decrease in number of platelets in the circulating blood.

thrombocytosis : increase in the number of platelets in the circulating blood.

Chapter 11
RESPIRATORY SYSTEM

Ⅰ. Respiratory system function

to provide the body tissues with oxygen and to remove carbon dioxide.

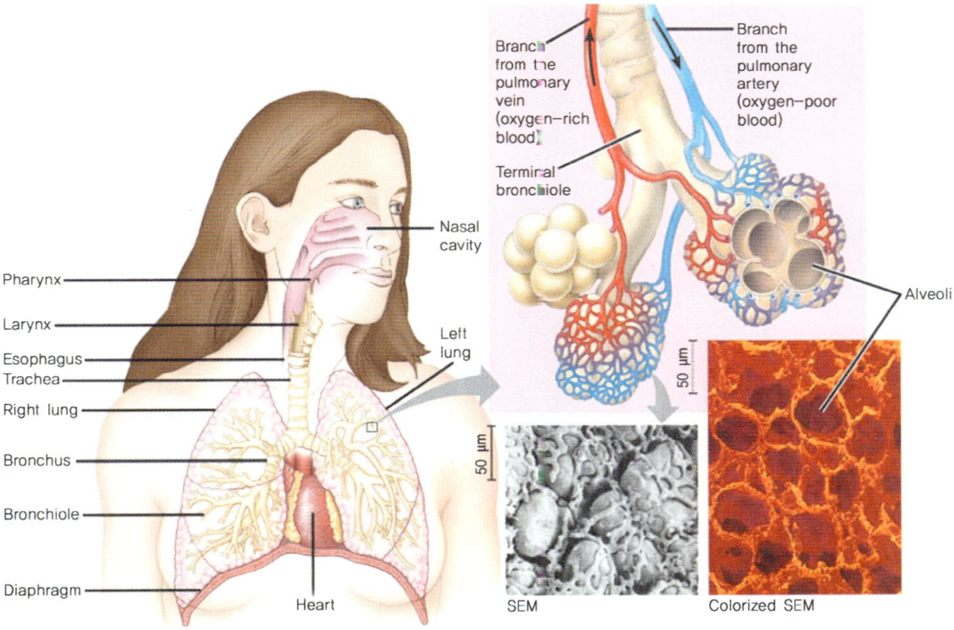

그림 11-1. Lungs and airways showing the structures through which air passes on its way to the lungs. Inset shows alveoli and capillaries.

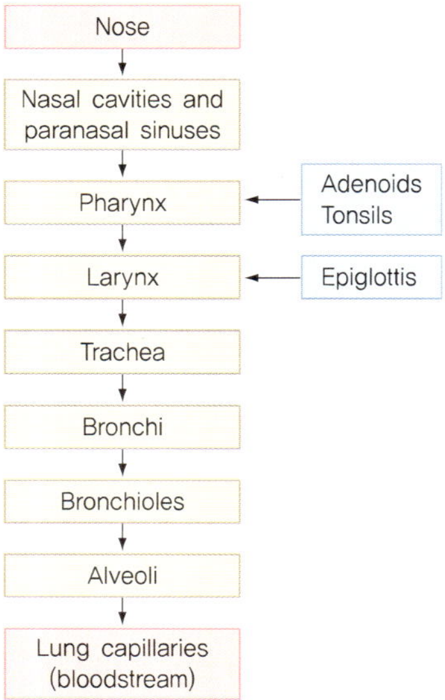

그림 11-2. Pathway of air from the nose to the capillaries of the lungs

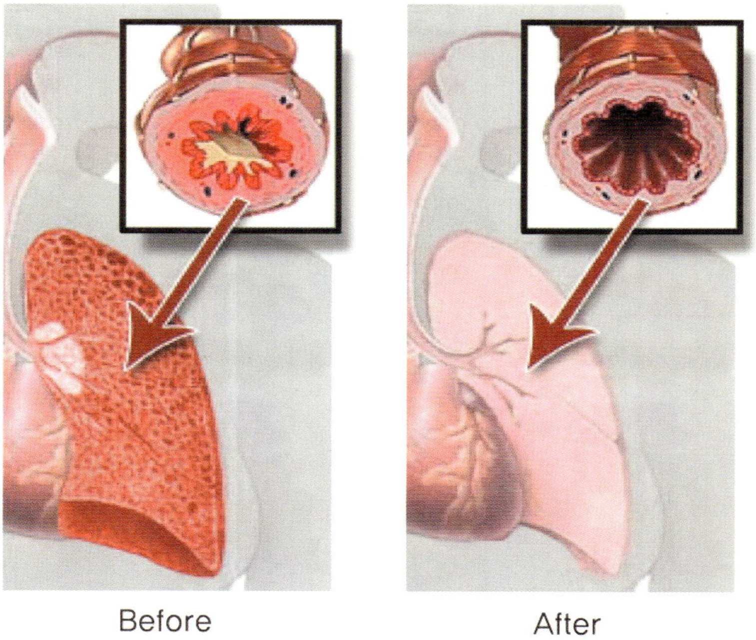

그림 11-3. Collapse

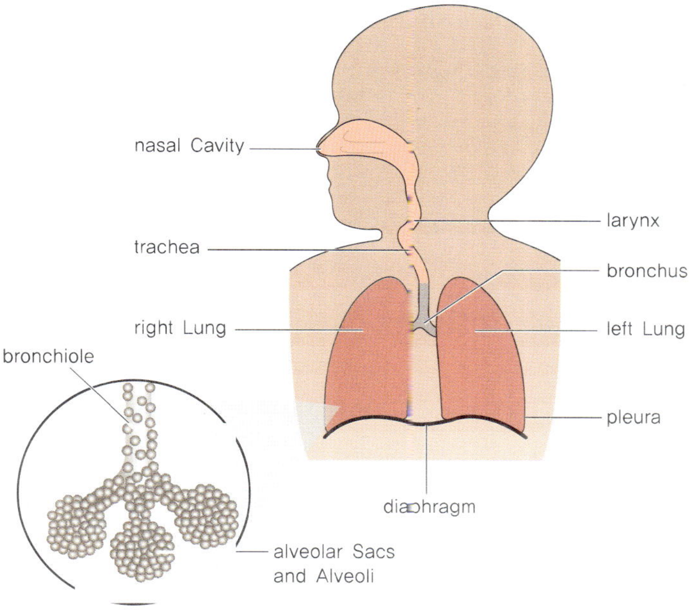

그림 11-4. Pneumonia

Ⅱ. Organs

nasal cavity : nose ; neres(naris is singular) ; nasal septum divides cavity.

pharynx : throat(through which air and food pass).

larynx : voice box ; vocal cords.

trachea : windpipe.

bronchi(bronchus) : one to each lung ; lined with cilia(hairlike projections).

bronchioles : smaller divisions of bronchi.

alveoli(alveolus) : tiny air sacs at the ends of bronchioles that comprise lung tissue. In the alveoli, the gaseous exchanges take place (oxygen picked up, carbon dioxide dropped off).

lungs : right, three lobes ; left, two lobes. Apex(a pices is plural) is the top of the lung ; the base is the bottom. They lie in the pleural cavity (thoracic cavity).

Respiration breathing ; consists of inspiration and expiration. Air enters the nasal cavity and oral cavity and travels through the preceding organs.
Diaphragm dome-shaped muscle that separates the pleural cavity from the abdominopelvic cavity. It moves downward on inspiration, creating suction in the chest to draw in air, expand lungs.

Ⅲ. Accessory structures

eustachian tubes : tubes from pharynx to middle ear, they equalize pressure.
epiglottis : flap that covers entrance to trachea ; it closes during swallowing to prevent aspiration of food.
inter costal muscles : muscles between ribs
paranasal sinuses : air spaces in cranium, connected to nasal cavity (frontal, maxillary, ethmoid, sphenoid).
pleura : double mucous membrane that covers the lungs(visceral layer) and lines the thoracic cavity(parietal layer).
tonsils and adenoids : part of the lymphatic system ; act as filters.
uvula : muscle tissue that hangs down from the soft palate ; it guards the opening from the nasal cavity, preventing food from entering ; staphyl/o=rootword for uvula ; for example, staphyloplasty.

Ⅳ. Function of the system

1. Word root

alveol/o	alveolus, air sac
antr/o, sin/o	antrum, sinus
bronch/o, bronchi/o	bronchial tube
bronchiol/o	bronchiole
laryng/o	voice box, larynx
nas/o, rhin/o	nose
osm/o	smell
pharyng/o	throat
phren/o	diaphragm
pleur/o	pleura
pne/o, spir/o	breathing
pneumon/o, pnenum/o	lung, air
pulmon/o	lung
thorac/o, steth/o	chest
tonsill/o	tonsils
trache/o	windpipe, trachea
turbin/o, conch/o	turbinate, concha

2. Anatomical terms

(1) Nose

choana	maxillary sinus
concha(pl, conchae)	meatus
ethmoid sinus	septum
external naris	sphenoidal sinus
frontal sinus	turbinate

(2) Pharynx

arytenoid cartilage	hyoid bone
auditary canal, Eustachian tube	laryngopharynx
corniculate cartilage	lingual tonsil
cricoid cartilage	nasopharynx
crypt	oropharynx
epiglottic cartilage	palatine tonsil
epiglottis	pharynx
fauces	thyroid cartilage
glottis	

(3) Trachea

apex pulmonis	lobe
alveolus	mediastinum
base of lung	parenchyma
bifurcation	segment
bronchiole	thorax
bronchus	trachea
hilus	

3. Medical terms

actinomycosis : an infection involving the deeper tissues of the skin and mucous membranes and caused by bacteria of the genus Actinomyces.

adenoidectomy : surgical excision of the adenoids. The operation is usually performed in conjunction with tonsillectomy since both the adenoids and palatine tonsils tend to become enlarged after repeated infections of the throat.

adenoiditis : inflammation of the adenoids.

adenoids : hypertrophy of the glandular tissue that normally exists in the nasopharynx of children and is known as the pharyngeal tonsil.

adenotonsillectomy : removal of the tonsils and adenoids.

allergic rhinitis : any allergic reaction of the nasal mucosa, occurring perennially(nonseasonal allergic rhinitis) or seasonally hay fever).

anosmia : absence of the sense of small.

anthracosis : a lung disease due to inhalation of coal dust not containing silica.

antrotomy : incision of antrum.

aphonia : loss of the voice; inability to produce vocal sounds.

apnea : temporary cessation of breathing.

asphyxia : a condition in which there is a deficiency of oxygen in the blood and an increase in carbon dioxide in the blood and tissues.

asthma : a condition marked by recurrent attacks of dyspnea, with wheezing due to spasmodic constriction of the bronchi.

atelectasis : a collapsed or airless state of the lung, which may be acute or chronic, and may involve all or part of the lung.

atresia of choana : congenital absence of paired opening between the nasal cavity and the nasopharynx.

atrophic rhinitis : chronic rhinitis with wasting of the mucous membrane and glands.

auscultation : the act of listening for sound within the body.

bradypnea, slow respiration : abnormal slowness of breathing.

bronchiectasis : chronic dilatation of the bronchi and bronchioles with secondary infection, usually involving the lower lobes of the lung.

bronchiolectasis : dilatation of the bronchioles.

bronchiolitis : inflammation of the bronchioles; bronchopneumonia.

bronchitis : inflammation of one or more bronchi.

bronchogenic carcinoma : carcinoma of the lung, so called because it arises from the epithelium of the bronchial tree.

bronchography : radiography of the bronchus after the injection of contrast material into the bronchus.

broncholithiasis : calculi in a part of the tracheobronchial tree.

bronchoscopy : inspection of the interior of the tracheobronchial tree through a bronchoscope. Bronchoscopy is used as a diagnostic aid and therapeutically.

bronchostenosis : stricture or cicatrical diminution of the bronchus.

bronchotomy : incision of a bronchus.

caldwell-luc operation : the operation of opening into the maxillary sinus by way of an incision into the supradental fossa opposite the premolar teeth.

chest radiography : a projection of the thoracic viscera shows the lungs, trachea, aorta, pulmonary regions.

cheyne-stokes respiration : breathing characterized by rhythmic waxing and waning of the depth of respiration; the patient breathes deeply for a short time and then breathes very slightly or stops breathing altogether.

congestion : excessive accumulation of blood.

cordectomy : excision of a vocal cord.

corditis : inflammation of vocal or spermatic cords.

coryza : profuse discharge from the mucous membrane of the nose.

croup : a condition resulting from acute obstruction of the larynx caused by allergy, foreign body, infection, or new growth, occurring chiefly in infants and children.

deviated nasal septum : The term septum is used to refer to the nasal septum, a plate of bone and cartilage covered with mucous membrane that divides the nasal cavity. An injury or malformation of this septum can produce a deviated septum, so that one part of the nasal cavity is smaller than the other. Occasionally the deviation may handicap breathing, block the normal flow of mucus from the sinuses during a cold, and prevent proper drainage of infected sinuses.

diphtheria : an acute, highly contagious childhood disease that generally affects the membranes of the throat and, less frequently, the nose, notably the skin, followeing an open wound, caused by the bacillus corynebacterium diphtheriae, it can be fatal if not treated promptly.

dysphagia : difficulty in swallowing.

dysphonia : any voice impairmint ; difficulty in speaking.

dyspnea : labored or difficult breathing.

effusion : escape of a fluid into a part ; exudation or transudation.

emphysema : a pathologic accumulation of air in tissues or organs. The term is generally used to designate chronic pulmonary emphysema, a lung disorder in which the terminal bronchioles become plugged with mucus.

epiglottitis : inflammation of epiglottis.

epistaxis : hemorrhage from the nose, usually due to rupture of small vessels overlying the anterior part of the cartilaginous nasal septum (Kiesselbachs area); nosebleed.

ethmoidectomy : excision of the ethmoid cells or of a portion of the ethmoid cell.

ethmoiditis : inflammation of the ethmoid bone or ethmoid sinuses.

eupnea : normal respiration.

exudate : a fluid with a high content of protein and cellular debris which has escaped from blood vessels and has been deposited in tissues or on tissue surfaces, usually as a result of inflammation.

friction rub : sound caused by the rubbing together of two serous surfaces.

hemoptysis : coughing and spitting of blood as a result of bleeding from any part of the respiratory tract. In true hemoptysis the sputum is bright red and frothy with air bubbles.

hemothorax : collection of blood in the pleural cavity.

hoarseness : a rough quality of voice.

hyaline membrane disease : a disorder of newborn infants, usually premature, characterized by the formation of a hyalin-like membrane lining the terminal respiratory passages.

hydrothorax : the presence of non inflammatory serous fluid within the pleural cavity.

hypercapnia, hypercarbia : excess of carbon dioxide in the circulating blood, with abnormally high carbon dioxide tension (Pco_2) causing overstimulation of respiratory center.

hypertrophic rhinitis : that with thickening and swelling of the mucous membrane.

hyperventilation : abnormally prolonged and deep breathing, usually associated with acute anxiety or emotional tension. It is most commonly seen in nervous, anxious females who have other functional disturbances related to emotional problem. A transient, respiratory alkalosis commonly results from hyperventilation. More proloned hyperventilation may be caused by disordors of the central nervous system, or by drugs, such as high concentration of salicylate, that increase the sensitivity of the respiratory centers.

hypoxia : oxygen want due to decreased amount of oxygen in organs and tissues.

laryngalgia : pain in the larynx.

laryngectomy : partial or total removal of the larynx by surgery.

laryngitis : inflammation of the larynx.

laryngography : radiography of the larynx after the injection of contrast medium into the larynx.

laryngoscopy : direct visual examination of the larynx with a laryngoscope.

lobectomy : excision of a lobe, as of the lung, or liver.

lung biopsy : the removal and examination, usually microscopic, of pulmonary tissue from the living body.

maxilloethmoidectomy : excision of the portion of the maxilla surrounding the maxillary sinus and of the cribriform plate and anterior ethmoid cells.

murmur : an auscultatory sound, benign or pathologic.

nasal polyps : focal accumulation of edema fluid in the nasal mucosa.

nasopharyngitis : inflammation of the nasopharynx.

orthopnea : ability to breathe easily only in the upright position.

paroxysm : a sudden recurrence or intensification of symptoms.

percussion : the act of striking a part with short.

peritonsillar abscess : a localized accumulation of pus in the peritonsillar tissue subsequent to supprative inflammation of the tonsil ; called also quinsy.

pertussis : an infectious disease due to Bordetella pertussis, and characterized by coryza, bronchitis, and a typical explosive cough ending in crowing or whooping inspiration.

pharyngalgia : pain in the pharynx.

pharyngitis : inflammation of the pharynx.

pharyngoplasty : plastic operation on the pharynx.

pleural effusion : the presence of liquid in the pleural space.

pleurectomy : excision of a portion of the pleura.

pleurisy, pleuritis : inflammation of the pleura ; it may be a complication of lung diseases, particularly of pneumonia, tuberculosis, lung abscess, or influenza.

pleurodynia : paroxymal pain in the intercostal muscles.

pneumoconiosis : any of a group of lung diseases resulting from inhalation of particles in the lungs.

pneumonectomy : excision of lung tissue, of an entire lung(total pneumonectomy) or less(partial pneumonectomy), or of a single lobe (lobectomy).

pneumonia : inflammation of the lung with consolidation and exudation.

pneumonitis : inflammation of lung tissue.

pneumothorax : accumulation of air or gas in the pleural cavity, resulting in collapse of the lung on the affected cavity.

polyp : any growth or mass protruding from a mucous membrane.

pulmonary edema : an effusion of serous fluid into the pulmonary interstitial tissues and air sacs.

pulmonary embolism : lodgment of a blood clot in a pulmonary artery with subsegunt obstruction of blood supply to the lung parenchyma.

pulmonary emphysema : enlargement of the air spaces.

pulmonary hypertension : increased pressure within the pulmonary circulation.

pulmanary infarction : hemorrhagic consolidation of lung parenchyma.

pulmonary tuberculosis : an infectious, inflammatory, reportable disease that is chronic in nature and commonly affects the lungs. The causative agent is the tubercle bacillus(Mycobascterium tuberculosis).

pyothorax : suppurative inflammation of the pleural space.

rales : an abnormal respiratory sound heard in auscultation and indicating some pathologic condition. Rales are distinguished as dry or moist, according to the absence or presence of fluid in the air passages.

rhinalgia, rhinodynia : pain in the nose.

rhinitis : inflammation of the mucous membrane of the nose.

rhinoplasty : plastic surgery of the nose.

rhinorrhea : the free discharge of a thin nasal mucus.

rhinotomy : incision into the nose.

rhonchus : a rattling in the throat ; also, a dry coarse rale in the bronchial tubes, due to a partial obstruction.

schick test : intracutaneous injection of diluted diphtheria toxin equal to one-fiftieth of the lethal dose. Lack of immunity to diphtheria is indicated by redness and edema at the injection site on the fifth to seventh day.

septal dermoplasty : dermoplasty of the nasal septum.

septectomy : excision of part of the nasal septum.

septoplasty : surgical reconstruction of the nasal septum.

siderosis : a form of pneumoconiosis due to the inhalation of iron or other metallic particles.

silicosis : a lung disease caused by the prolonged inhalation of silica.

sinusitis : inflammation of one or more of the paranasal sinuses, often occurring during an upper respiratory infection, when infection in the nose spreads to the sinuses.

sneeze : to expel air forcibly throuth the nose and mouth.

stridor : a shrill, harsh sound, especially the respiratory sound heard during inspiration in laryngeal obstruction.

tachypnea : excessive rapidity of respiration.

thoracentesis : surgical puncture and drainage of the thoracic cavity.

thoracoplasty : surgical removal of ribs, allowing the chest wall to collapse a diseased lung.

thoracoscopy : examination of the pleura through a scope under general anesthesia.

thoracotomy : incision of the chest wall.

tonsillectomy : excision of tonsils, The procedure is performed in treament of chronic infection of the tonsils.

tonsillitis : inflammation and enlargement of a tonsil, especially the palatine tonsils.

tracheitis : inflammation of the trachea.

tracheobronchitis : inflammation of the trachea and bronchi.

tracheoesophageal fistula : most commonly a fistula from near the carina of the trachea to the lower esophageal segment.

tracheoplasty : a plastic operation upon the trachea.

tracheorrhagia : hemorrhage from the trachea.

tracheostenosis : contraction or narowing of the trachea.

tracheostomy : creation of an opening into the trachea through the neck, with insertion of an indwelling tube to facilitate passage of air or evacuation of secretions.

tracheotomy : incision of trachea through the skin and muscles of the neck for exploration, for removal of a foreign body, or for obtaining a biopsy specimen or removing a local lesion.

transudate : a fluid substance that has passed through a membrane or has been extruded from a tissue; in contrast to an exudate, a transudate is characterized by high fluidity and a low content of protein, cells, or solid matter derived from cells.

turbinectomy : excision of a turbinate bone(nasal concha).

Chapter

12 MUSCULOSKELETAL SYSTEM

Ⅰ. Musculoskeletal system

Functions

1. Supports and gives shape to body.
2. Protects internal organs.
3. Makes movement possible.
4. Forms blood cells(in red bone marrow, long bones).

Skeleton the following are the main divisions :

1. Axial : skull, thorax(ribs and sternum), vertebral column.
2. Appendicular : the appendages that hang from the axial skeleton ; upper and lower extremities(includes shoulder and pelvic girdle).

Large bones of the body

clavicle : collar bone.

sternum : breast bone.

humerus : upper arm.

radius and ulna : forearm.

femur : thigh(longest bone in the body).

fibula and tibia : lower leg.

scapula : shoulder blade.

vertebral column : starting at the neck : cervical vertebrae(7), thoracic or dorsal(12), lumbar(5), sacral(5, fused), coccyx or tail bone(4).

cranial bones(also called skull or calvaria)

frontal : forehead(1).

parietal : top of head(2).

temporal : temples(2).

occipital : back of head(1).

ethmoid : upper nasal, between eyes(1).

sphenoid : behind eyes(base of skull), and laterally between parietal and temporal bones(1).

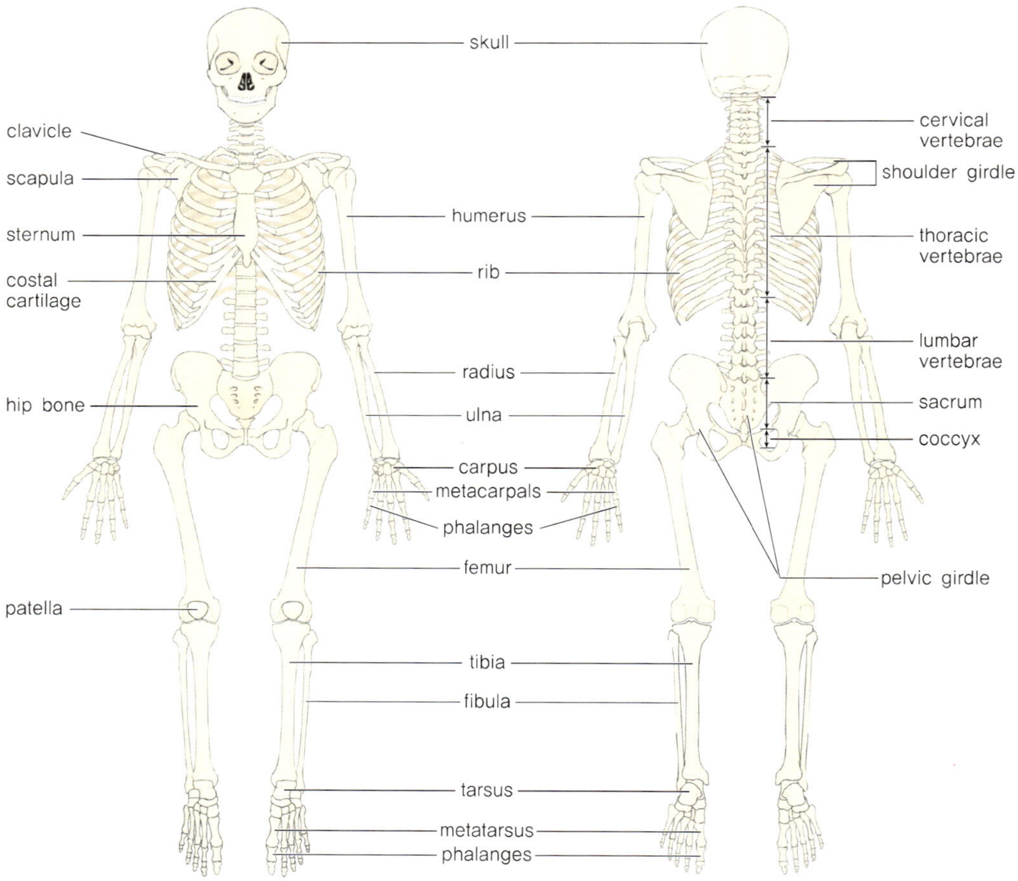

그림 12-1. Skeleton. Left, anterior view, showing large bones of the body. Right, posterior view, showing large bones and sections of vertebral column.

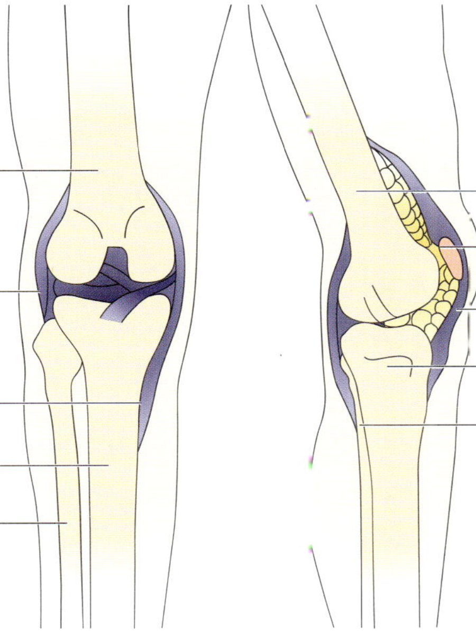

그림 12-2. Knee, anterolateral aspect, with synovial asc and adjacent bursae. Shows large bones of the leg, some tendons and ligaments.

mandible : lower jaw(1).

maxilla : upper jaw(2).

turbinates : cone-shaped nasal bones(2).

malar : cheekbones(2) ; also called zygomatic.

Ⅱ. Joints and related structures

(articulations) hold bones securely.

aponeurosis : flattened tendon ; resembles a membrane.

ball and socket joint : hip and shoulder joints.

bursa(ae) : small sacs that serve to cushion joints ; between tendons and bones.

fascia(ae) : connective tissue sheath ; holds muscle fibers together ; covers, supports and separates muscles.

hinge joint : elbows, knees, fingers.

interphalangeal joints : fingers and toes ; DIP is distal interphalangeal and PIP is proximal interphalangeal.
intervertebral disks(discs) : cartilaginous substance between vertebrae.
lamina(ae) : the flattened part of the vertebral arch(thinnest part of a vertebra).
ligament : strong fibrous tissue connecting bone to bone.
meniscus(ci) : cartilage of the knee, lateral and medial, on the superior surface of the tibia(articulates with femur).
sutures : articulations in the cranial bones ; immovable joints.
synovial fluid : clear fluid present in joints(lubrication).
temporomandibular joint(TMJ) : junction of lower jaw bone and temporal bone.
tendon : fibrous tissue attaching muscle to bone.
theca : covering or sheath of a tendon.

Skeletal differences female skeleton has a wider pelvis. The infant skeleton has a larger head(for the size of its body), consists partly of cartilage so is softer than adults, and infant skull bones have spaces between them (fontanels or soft spots).

Ⅲ. Terms used to describe projections, openings, and indentations in bones

acetabulum : large socket for head of femur(hip).
foramen(pl. foramina) : holes in a bone for large vessels and nerves to pass through, for example, foramen magnum.
fossa(ae) : depressions or hollows.
grooves : shallow linear depressions in bone(or tooth).
malleolus : hammerlike protuberance(either side of ankle).

olecranon : a process on the ulnar bone(elbow).

prominences, processes, tuberosities : projections.

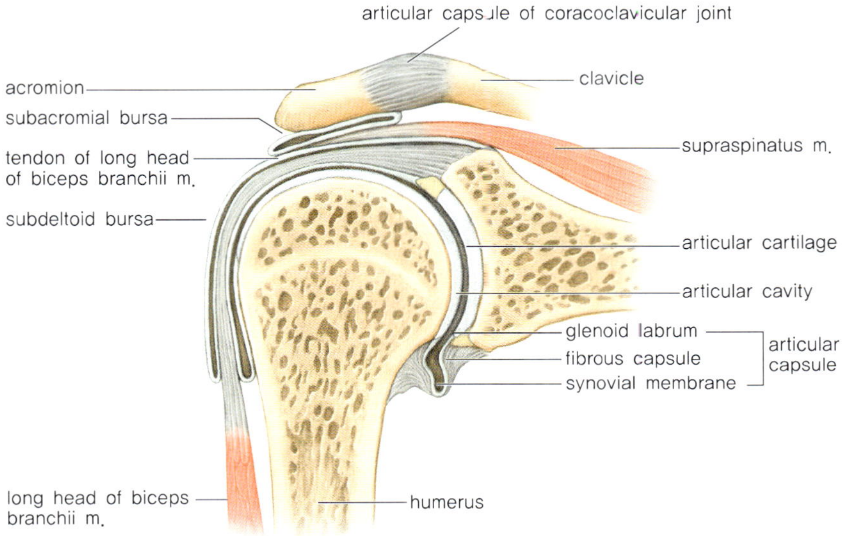

그림 12-3. Bony tissue

sinuses : air spaces in cranium that make the skull lighter and serve as resonating chambers for the voice. (sinus has some other meanings.)

Names of the small bones of the ankle, foot, and wrist are not given in this text. Should you need these, most medical dictionaries list bones in the appendix. Tabers dictionary lists them under skeleton. Similar lists of muscles, joints, ligaments, and so on are also usually given in the appendix of medical dictionaries.

Muscles there are three kinds of muscle tissue :

1. Striated(striped appearance) ; also called skeletal muscle (voluntary).
2. Nonstriated : smooth muscle. Called involuntary as we have no control over it. Causes peristaltic movement of stomach and intestines.

3. Cardiac muscle : heart muscle.

Skeletal muscles are attached to two bones(origin and insertion) and are joined together by a movable joint. Skeletal muscles are attached by tendons. The largest tendon is the Achilles tendon ; originates from calf muscles, insertion to calcaneus(heel bone).

Ⅳ. Function of the system

1. Word root

arthr/o, articul/o	joint
brachi/o	arm
chondr/o	cartilage
cost/o	rib
digit/o, dactyl/o	finger, toe
dors/o	dorsum
gnath/o	jaw
leiomy/o	smooth, visceral muscle
ligament/o, syndesm/o	ligaments
man/o	hand
ment/o	mentum, chin
my/o, myos/o	muscle
myel/o	bone marrow
oste/o	bone
plant/o	foot sole
ped/o, pod/o	foot
rhabdomy/o	skeletal, striated muscle
sarc/o	flesh
spin/o, rachi/o	spinal column, vertebrae
ten/o, tend/o, tendin/o	tendons
vertebr/o, spondyl/o	vertebrae

2. Anatomical terms

(1) Cranium

anterior or bregmatic fontanelle	nasal bone
cranium	occipital bone
ethmoid bone	palatine bone
foramen magnum	parietal bone
frontal bone	posterior or occipital fontanelle
hyoid bone	sphenoid bone
lacrimal bone	temporal bone
mandible	vomer
maxilla	zygomatic bone

(2) Vertebrae

atlas	lumbar vertebrae
cervical vertebrae	rib
cervical curvature	sacrum
coccyx	sternum
costal cartilage	thoracic curvature
false ribs	thoracic vertebrae
floating ribs	thorax
intervertabral disk	true ribs, vertebrosternal ribs
lumbar curvature	

(3) Extremity

acetabulum	patella
carpal bone	phalanx(pl. phalanges)
clavicle	radius
femur	scapula
fibula	tarsal bone
humerus	tibia
metacarpal bone	ulna
metatarsal bone	

(4) Hip bone

acetabulum	pelvic outlet
false pelvis	pelvis
hip bone	pubic arch
ilium	pubis
ischium	true pelvis
pelvic inlet	

(5) Articulation and muscle

aponeurosis	smooth muscle
articular capsule	striated muscle
articulation	synovia
involuntary muscle	tendon
ligament	voluntary muscle
skeletal muscle	

3. Medical terms

amelia : a developmental anomaly with abscence of the limbs.

anencephalia : absence of the cranial vault.

arthralgia : pain in a joint.

arthrocentesis : puncture and aspiration of a joint.

arthroscopy : examination of the interior of a joint with an arthroscope.

bone graft : a piece of bone used to take the place of a removed bone or bony defect.

chondrectomy : excision of the cartilage.

chondroma : a tumor of cartilage cells.

chondromalacia : abnormal softening of cartilage.

chondrotomy : the dissection or the surgical division of cartilage.

closed fracture : fracture that does not produce an open wound, simple fracture.

colle's fracture : fracture of the lower end of the radius, the distal fragment being displaced backward.

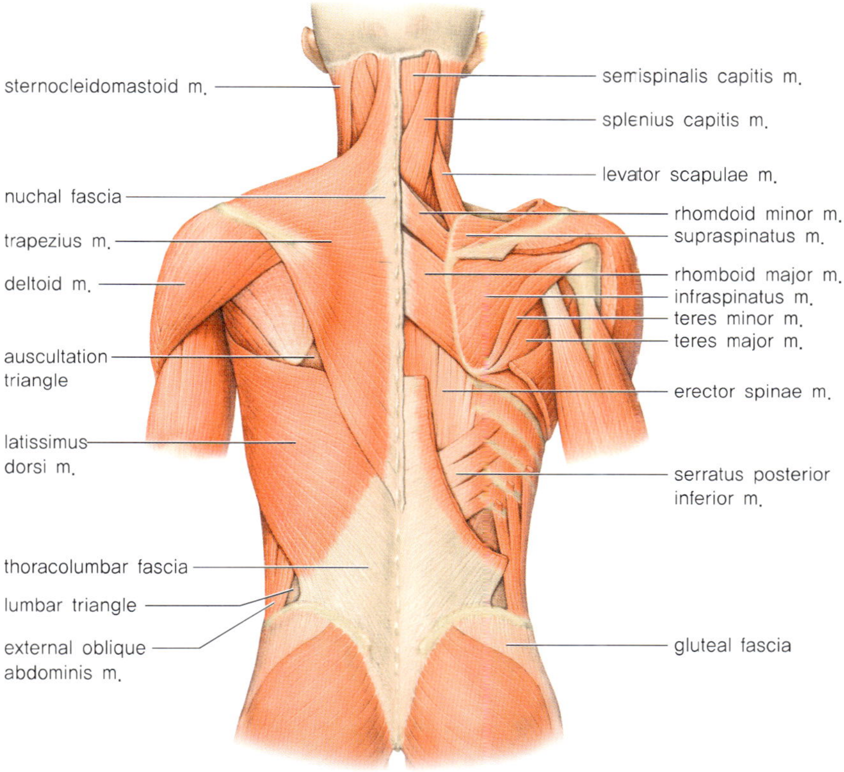

그림 12-4. Shoulder dissection from rear (muscles, tendons fascia, and bursa)

comminuted fracture : fracture in which the bone is splintered or crushed.

compression fracture : fracture produced by compression.

coxa valga : deformity of the hip joint with increase in the angle of inclination between the neck and shaft of the femur.

coxa vara : deformity of the hip joint with decrease in the angle of inclination between the neck and shaft of the femur.

cramp : a painful spasmodic muscular contraction.

craniomalacia : abnormal softness of the bones of the skull.

craniostosis : congenital ossification of the cranial sutures.

crepitation : a dry, crackling sound or sensation, such as that produced by the grating of the ends of a fractured bone.

depressed fracture : fracture of the skull in which a fragment is depressed.

dislocation : displacement of a bone from a joint. The most common dislocations are those involving a finger, thumb, or shoulder.

electromyography : recording the electrical activity evoked in a muscle by electrical stimulation.

ewing's tumor : a malignant tumor of the bone arising in medullary tissue.

exostosis : a benign bony growth projecting outward from the surface of a bone.

fracture : the breaking of a part, especially bone.

genu valgum : a deformity in which the knees are abnormally close together and the space between the ankles is increased.

genu varum : bow leg.

greenstick fracture : fracture in which one side of a bone is broken, the other being bent.

kyphosis : increased convexity in the curvature of the thoracic spine as viewed from the side; called also hunchback.

hallux valgus : angulation of the great toe toward the other toes of the foot.

hallux varus : angulation of the great toe away from the other toes of the foot.

hemathrosis : blood in a joint cavity.

hammer toe : a condition in which the proximal phalanx of the toe is extended and the second and distal phalanges are flexed, causing a clawlike appearance.

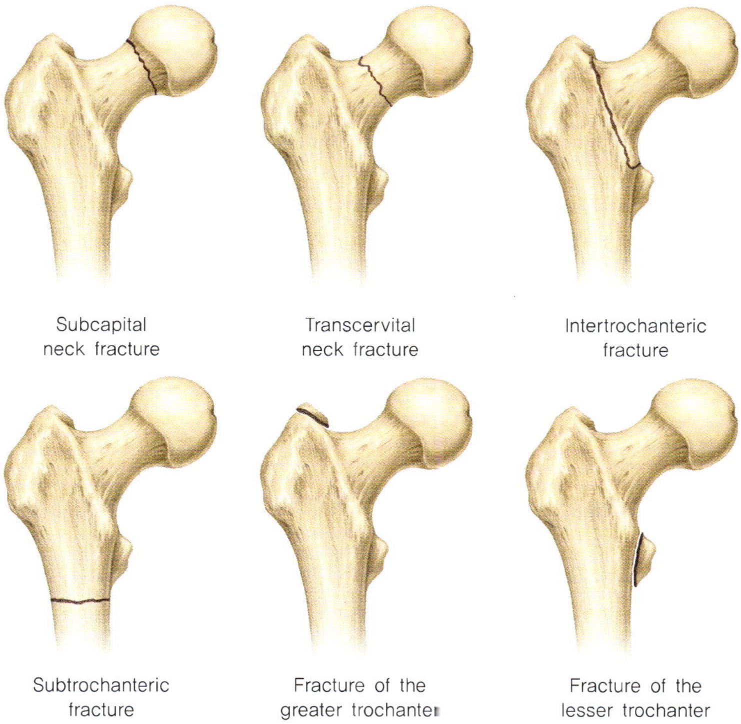

그림 12-5. Examples of some types of fractures

herniation : abnormal protrusion of an organ or other body structure through a defect or natural opening in a covering membrane, muscle or bone.

herniation of nucleus pulposus : rupture or prolapse of the nucleus pulposus into the spinal canal, or against the spinal cord.

hydrathrosis : an accumulation of watery fluid in the cavity of a joint.

hyperkinesia : abnormally increased motor function or activity.

hypophosphatasia : an inborn error of metabolism, characterized by lowered phosphatase activity of the serum.

incomplete fracture : fracture that does not involve the complete cross section of the bone.

impacted fracture : fracture in which one fragment is firmly driven into the other.

knee arthrography : radiography of knee joint after injection of contrast material into the patellofemoral joint.

kocher's operation : a method of excising the ankle joint by a cut.

laminectomy : surgical excision of the posterior arch of a vertebrae during laminectomy the spinal cord is exposed and the portion of the nucleus pulposus that has herniated through the ruptured disk is removed.

lordosis : forward curvature of the lumbar spine.

lumbago : pain in the lower part of the back.

lund's operation : removal of the astragalus for the correction of a talipes.

multiple myeloma : a malignant neoplasm of plasma cell arising in the bone marrow.

muscle biopsy : removal and examination, usually microscopic, of muscular tissue from the living body.

nonunion : failure of the ends of a fractured bone to unit.

open fracture : fracture in which a wound through the adjacent or overlying soft tissues communicates with the site of the break.

ostealgia : pain in the bones, osteodynia.

ostectomy : excision of a bone or part of a bone.

osteitis, ostitis : inflammation of a bone.

osteocamp : an instrument for bending the femur.

osteochondritis : inflammation of both bone and cartilage.

osteochondroma : a benign tumor consisting of projecting adult bone capped by cartilage.

osteoclasis : surgical fracture or refracture of a bone.

osteodysplasty : abnormal development of bone.

osteodystrophy : defective bone formation.

osteoma : a tumor composed of bone tissue.

osteomyelitis : inflammation of bone caused by a pyogenic organism.

osteoplasty : plastic surgery of the bones.

osteoporosis : abnormal rarefaction of bone ; the principal causes are lack of physical activity, lack of estrogen or androgens, nutritional deficiency, and aging. Symptoms include pathologic fractures and collapse of the vertebrae without compression of the spinal cord.

osteosarcoma : a osteogenic sarcoma.

osteotomoclasis : correction of curvature of bone by partial division with the osteotome.

pathologic fracture : fracture due to weakening of the bone structure by pathologic processes, such as neoplasia, osteomalacia, or osteomyelitis.

pott's disease : tuberculosis of the spine, usually beginning as a tuberculous osteomyelitis of the vertabrae and progressing to damage of the intervertebral disks symptoms include stiffness of the back, pain on motion, prominence of the spinous process of certain vertebrae and occasionally abscess formation.

pott's fracture : fracture of lower part of fibula with serious injury of the lower tibial articulation.

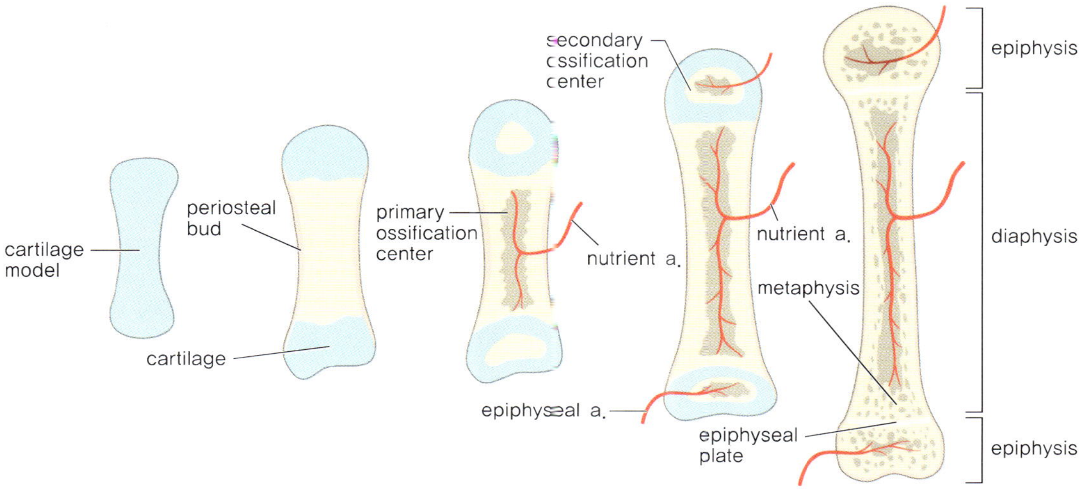

그림 12-6. Ossification

reduction : the correction of a fracture, luxation, or hernia.

rheumatoid arthritis : a chronic disease marked by inflammatory changes in the synovial membrane and articular strutures.

rickets : a condition of infancy and childhood caused by deficiency of vitamin D, which leads to altered calcium and phosphorus metabolism and consequent disturbance of ossification of bone.

scoliosis : lateral deviation in the normally straight vertical line of the spine ; it may not include rotation or deformity of the vertebrae.

scurvy : deficiency of vitamin C in the diet.

sequestrum : a piece of dead that has become separated during the process of necrosis from sound bone.

spasm : a sudden involuntary contraction of a muscle or group of muscle.

spina bifida : defective closure of the bony encasement of the spinal cord.

spiral fracture : the bone has been twisted apart.

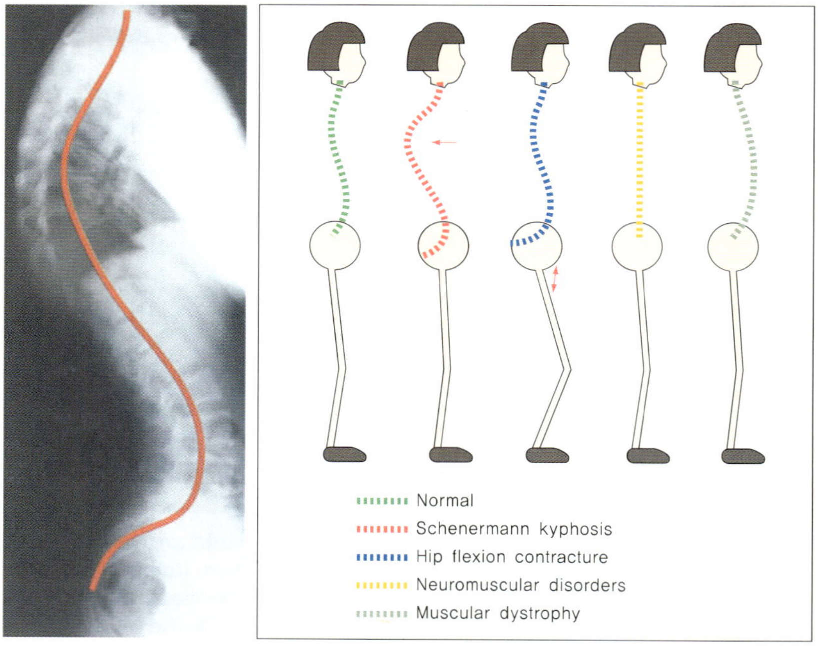

그림 12-7. Musculoskeletal deformities

spondylitis : inflammation of the vertebra.

sprain : wrenching or twisting of a joint, with partial rupture of its ligament.

strain : to overexercise, an overstretching or overexertion of some part of the musculature.

subluxation : incomplete or partial dislocation.

synarthrosis : a form of a articulation united by continuous fibrous tissue.

syndactylia : the most common congenital anomaly of the hand, marked by the persistence of the webbing between adjacent digits, so they are more or less completely attached. The anomaly may also occur in the foot.

talipes : a congenital deformity of the foot, clubfoot ; the foot may have an abnormally high longitudinal arch(talipes cavus), or it may be in dorsiflexion(talipes calcaneus) or plantar flexion(talipes equinus), abducted & everted(talipes valgus), abducted & inverted(talipes varus).

transverse fracture : a fracture at right angles to the axis of the bone.

Chapter

13 ENDOCRINE SYSTEM

I. Endocrine system

Function to regulate body activity and, together with the nervous system, help maintain homeostasis.

All of the organs in the endocrine system are glands.

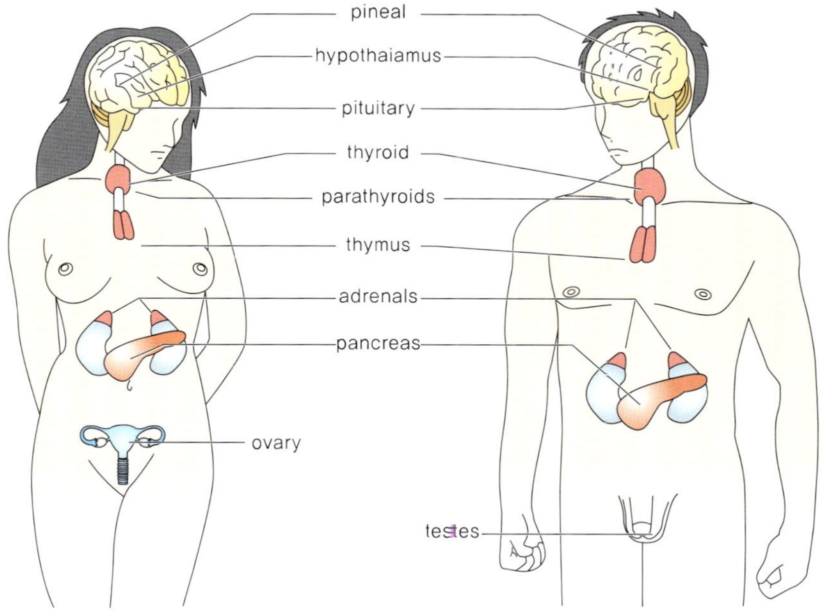

그림 13-1. Endocrine glands, small but very important ductless glands that secrete hormones directly into the bloodstream. Hormones produced are shown in parentheses.

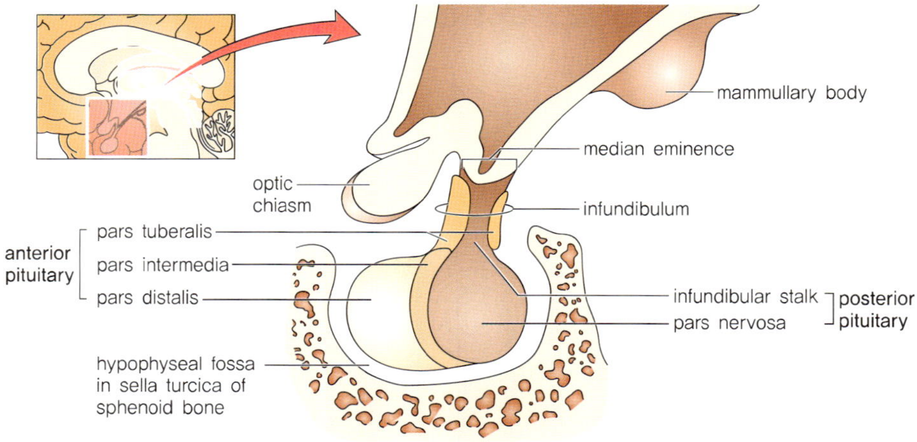

그림 13-2. Pituitary gland

They are called ductless glands(or glands of internal secretion) because they have no ducts. (A duct is a narrow tube that carries secretions.)

Ductless glands secrete hormones internally, directly into the blood stream, instead of into ducts. Hormones affect many body functions.

endocrine glands : Location, Function

pituitary(hypophysis ; anterior and posterior) : deep in cranial cavity ; called master gland, as it affects all others.

thyroid(shaped "like a shield") : aside and in front of larynx(neck) ; alters metabolic rate and secretes thyroxine(high in iodine).

parathyroids(four) : behind thyroid ; regulate calcium and phosphorus content of blood and bones.

adrenals(cortex, outer ; medulla, inner) : one atop each kidney ; secrete steroids(corticoids) and help body cope with stress.

pancreas : behind stomach ; controls use of sugar and starch. Islands of Langerhans secrete insulin (beta cells).

sex glands(gonads) : ovaries secrete estrogens and progesterone ; testes secrete testosterone.

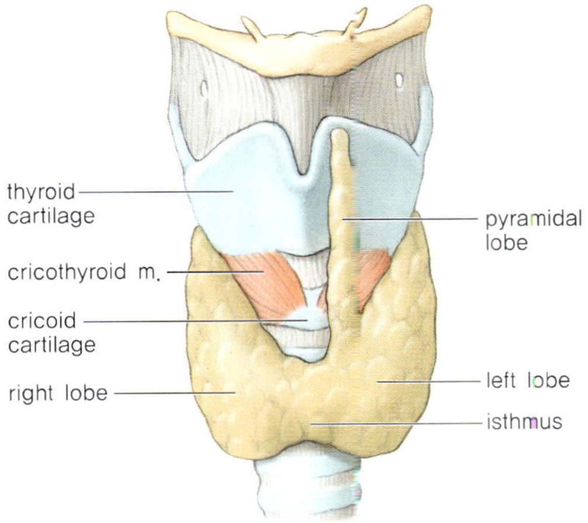

그림 13-3. Ventral view of thyroid gland

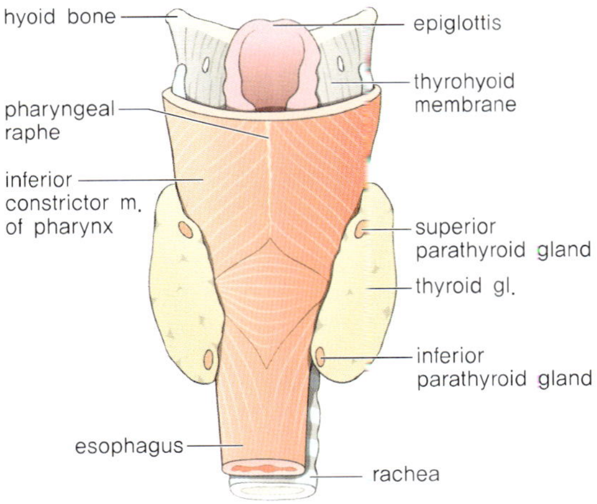

그림 13-4. Dorsal view of parathyroid glands

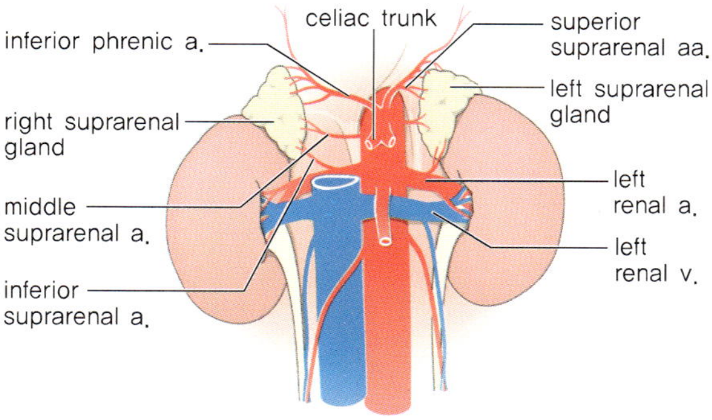

그림 13-5. The adrenal glands

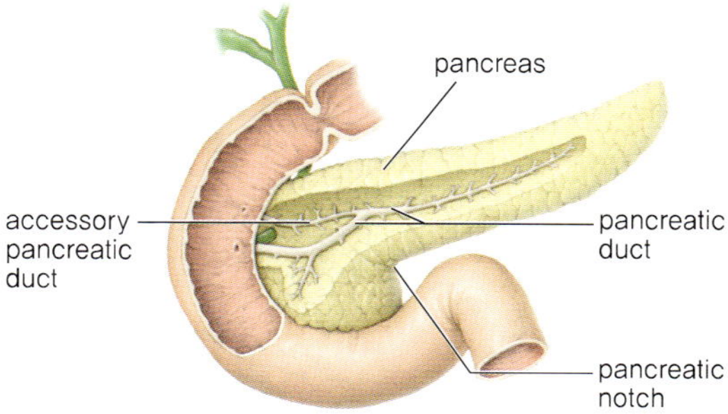

그림 13-6. Pancreas

pineal gland : base of brain(little is known about it).

thymus : pleural cavity(mediastinum) ; decreases in size in adult(may have some function in immune responses).

Ⅱ. Function of the system

1. Word root

adren/o, adrenal/o	adrenal gland
crin/o	secretion
gigant/o	huge
glyc/o, gluc/o	sugar
immun/o	immune
lact/o, galact/o	milk
myx/o	mucus
parathyroid/o	parathyroid gland
pineal/o	pineal body
somat/o	body
thym/o	thymus gland
thyroid/o, thyr/o	thyroid gland

2. Anatomical terms

adrenal gland	pineal body
endocrine gland	pituitary gland, hypophysis
exocrine gland	testis
ovary	thymus gland
pancreas	thyroid gland
parathyroid gland	

3. Medical terms

acromegaly : abnormal enlargement of the extremities of the skeleton nose, jaws, hands, and feet resulting from hypersecretion of growth hormone from pituitary gland.

addison's disease : a syndrome resulting from insufficient production of hormones from the cortex of the adrenal gland(glucocorticoids and mineral corticoids).

adrenalectomy : surgical excision of an adrenal gland. This procedure is indicated when a disorder of the adrenal gland, such as Cushing's syndrome.

adrenogenital syndrome : hyperfunction of the adrenal cortex.

aldosteronism : an abnormality of electrolyte balance caused by excessive secretion-of aldosterone; called also aldosteronism.

basedow's disease : exophthalmic goiter.

crenitism : arrested physical and mental development with dystrophy of bones and soft tissues, due to congenital lack of thyroid gland secretion from hypofunctioning or absence of the gland.

cushing's syndrome : a group of symptoms produced by an excess of free circulating cortisol from the adrenal cortex. The symptoms and signs include painful fatty swellings in the interscapular area(buffalo hump) and in the facial area(moon face), distention of the abdomen, ecchymoses following even minor trauma, impotence, amenorrhea, high blood pressure, and loss of muscle mass. There also can be an unusual growth of body hair in females(hirsutism) and streaked purple markings(atrophic striae) in the abdominal area as a result of collections of body fat.

dehydration : the condition that result from excessive loss of body water.

diabetes : a general form referring to a variety of disorders characterized by excessive urination(polyuria), as in diabetes mellitus and diabetes insipidus.

diabetes insipidus : a disorder characterized by a urinary output of from 2 to 10 liters per day, and an increased intake of fluid that does not match the output.

diabetes mellitus : a broadly applied term used to denote a complex group of syndromes that have in common a disturbance on the oxidation and utilization of glucose, which is secondary to a malfunction of the beta cells of the pancreas, whose function is the production and release of insulin.

dietotherapy : treatment of the diabetes mellitus by regulation of the diet.

dwarfism : the state of being a dwarf ; under development of the body.

exophthalmos : abnormal protrusion of the eye.

froehlich's syndrome : a condition associated with lesions of the hypothalamus and pituitary gland, marked by obesity and sexual infantilism ; called also adiposogenital dystrophy.

gigantism : abnormal overgrowth of the body or a part ; excessive size and stature.

glucosuria : the presence of glucose in the urine.

goiter : enlargement of the thyroid gland, causing a swelling in the front part of the neck. Simple endemic goiter is usually caused by lack of iodine in the diet. Exophthalmic, or toxic, goiter is accompanied by excessive concentrations of thyroid hormones in the blood, which produce the symptoms of hyperthyroidism.

graves disease : a clinical syndrome in which thyrotoxicosis is associated with diffuse goiter, infiltrative exophthalmos, and sometimes infiltrative dermopathy.

hirsutism : abnormal hairiness, especially in women.

hyperadrenocorticism, hyperadrenocorticalism : hypersecretion of the adrenal cortex ; Cushing's syndrome.

hyperglycemia : abnormally increased content of sugar in the blood.

hyperparathyroidism : abnormally increased activity of the parathyroid gland which may be primary or secondary.

hyperpituitarism : a condition due to pathologically increased activity of the pituitary gland, especially increased secretion of growth hormone, resulting in acromegaly or gigantism.

hypoadrenalism : deficiency of adrenal activity, as in Addisons disease.

hypoglycemia : an abnormally diminished content of glucose in the blood.

hypothyroidism : deficiency of thyroid gland activity, with under-production of thyroxine, or the condition resulting from it.

hypoparathyroidism : the condition produced by greatly reduced function of the parathyroid glands or by the removal of these bodies.

hypophysectomy : excision of the hypophysis, or pituitary gland.

hypopituitarism : the condition resulting from diminution or cessation of hormonal secretion by the pituitary gland, especially the anterior pituitary.

myxedema : a condition resulting from advanced hypothyroidism, or deficiency of thyroxine. It is the adult form of the disease known as cretinism in its congenital form.

osteitis fibrosa cystica : rarefying osteitis with fibrous degeneration and the formation of cysts and the presence of fibrous nodules on the affected bones, due to osteoclastic activity secondary to hyperparathyroidism.

palpitation : an unduly rapid or irregular heart beat.

parathyroidectomy : excision of a parathyroid gland.

pheochromocytoma : vascular tumor of the adrenal medulla.

pinealoblastoma : pinealoma in which the pineal cells are not well differentiated.

progeria : premature old age, a condition occurring in childhood marked by small stature, absence of facial and pubic hair, wrinkled skin, and eventual development of atherosclerosis.

simmonds disease : panhypopituitarism in which cachexia is a prominent feature; called also pituitary cachexia. It follows the destruction of the pituitary gland by surgery, infection, injury, or tumor.

tetany : continuous tonic spasm of a muscle. It is due to abnormal calcium metabolism, and occurs in parathyroid hypofunction, vitamin D deficiency and alkalosis.

thymectomy : excision of the thymus.

thymoma : a tumor derived from the epithelial or lymphoid elements of the thymus.

thyroidectomy : surgical excision of the thyroid gland.

thyrotoxicosis, Basedow's disease : a condition resulting from overactivity of the thyroid gland.

virilism : the presence of male characteristics in the female.

Chapter 14

INTEGUMENTARY SYSTEM

Ⅰ. Functions of skin

protection : a waterproof overcoat that keeps body fluids in and harmful elements out(bacteria and sun, for example).

sensory organ(receptor) : for sensations of touch, pain and temperature.

temperature regulator : for cooling and heating(perspiration and goose flesh).

waste elimination : disposal of wastes.

skin : integument(from Latin, meaning a covering), or external covering.

epidermis(cuticle) : non-vascular outer layer of skin ; consists of four **layers** : epithelial tissue. Cells on the surface are deal cells.

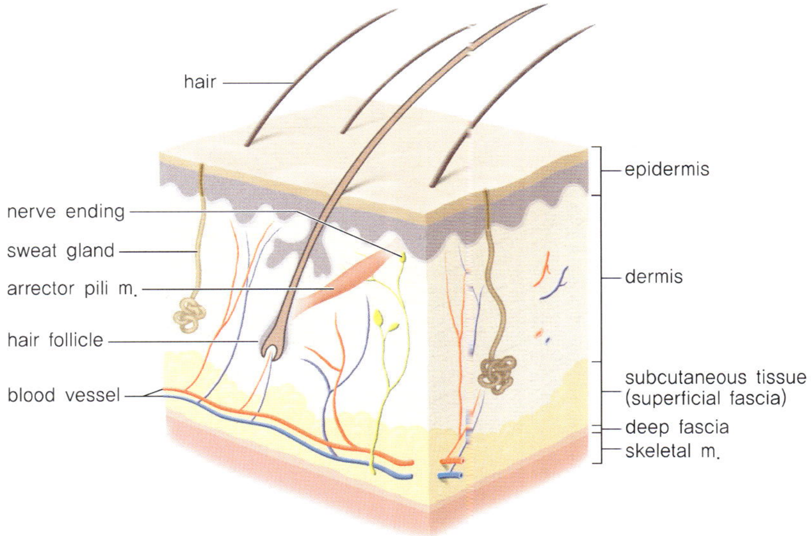

그림 14-1. Cross section of normal skin showing epidermis, dermis (corium) and subcutaneous tissues. Note important structures in dermis : blood vessels, sweat glands, and sebaceous glands.

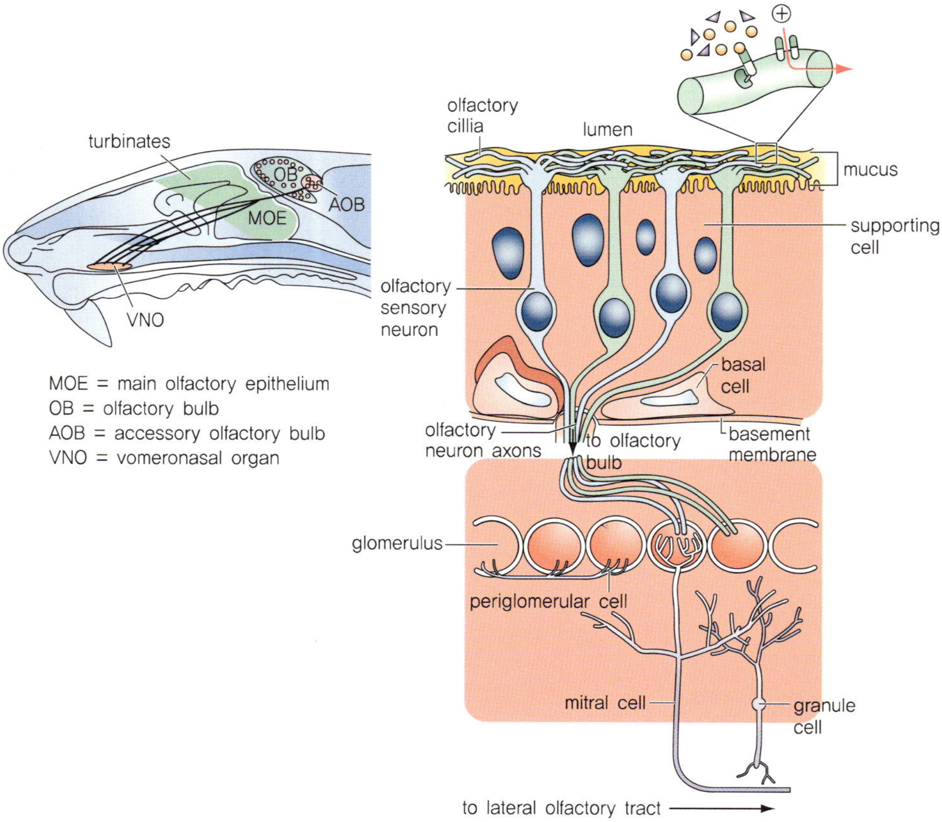

그림 14-2. Accessory organs of the skin

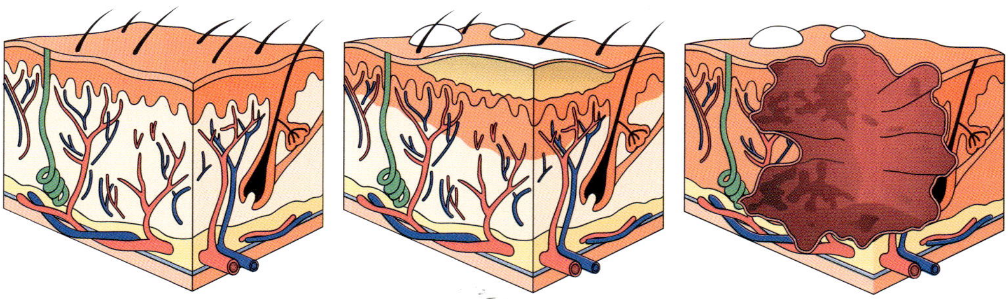

First Degree Burn
Involves top layers of epidermis only

Second Degree Burn
- Skin blisters
- involves sall of epidermis and some of dermis
- May involve all of dermis

Third Degree Burn
May extend into deeper tissues

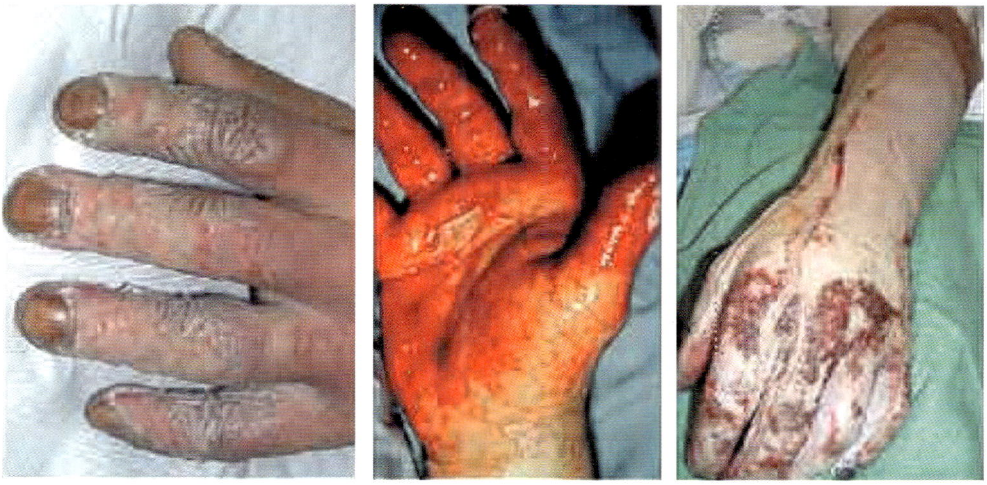

그림 14-3. Classificati□n of burns

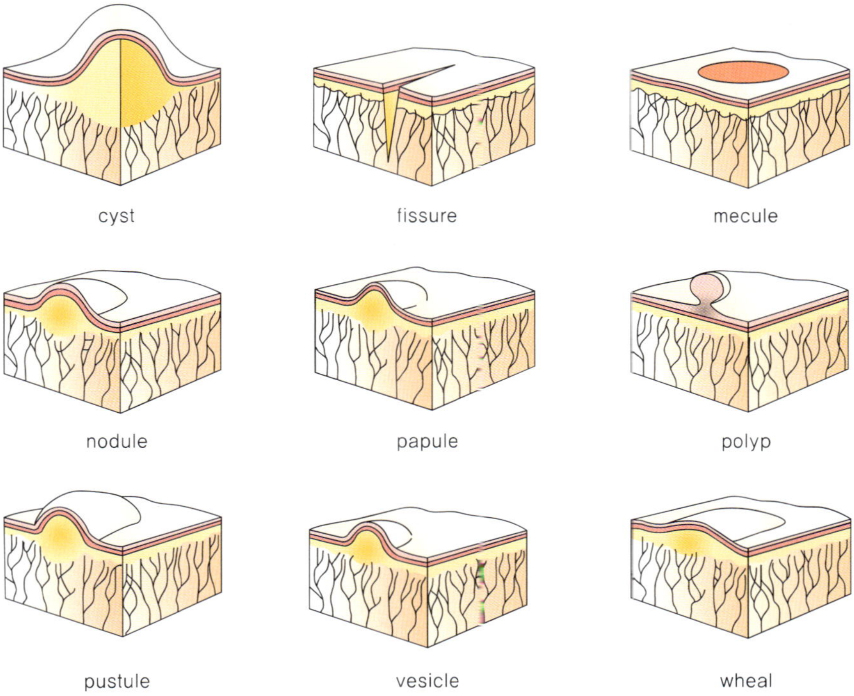

그림 14-4. Types of skin lesions—primary lesions

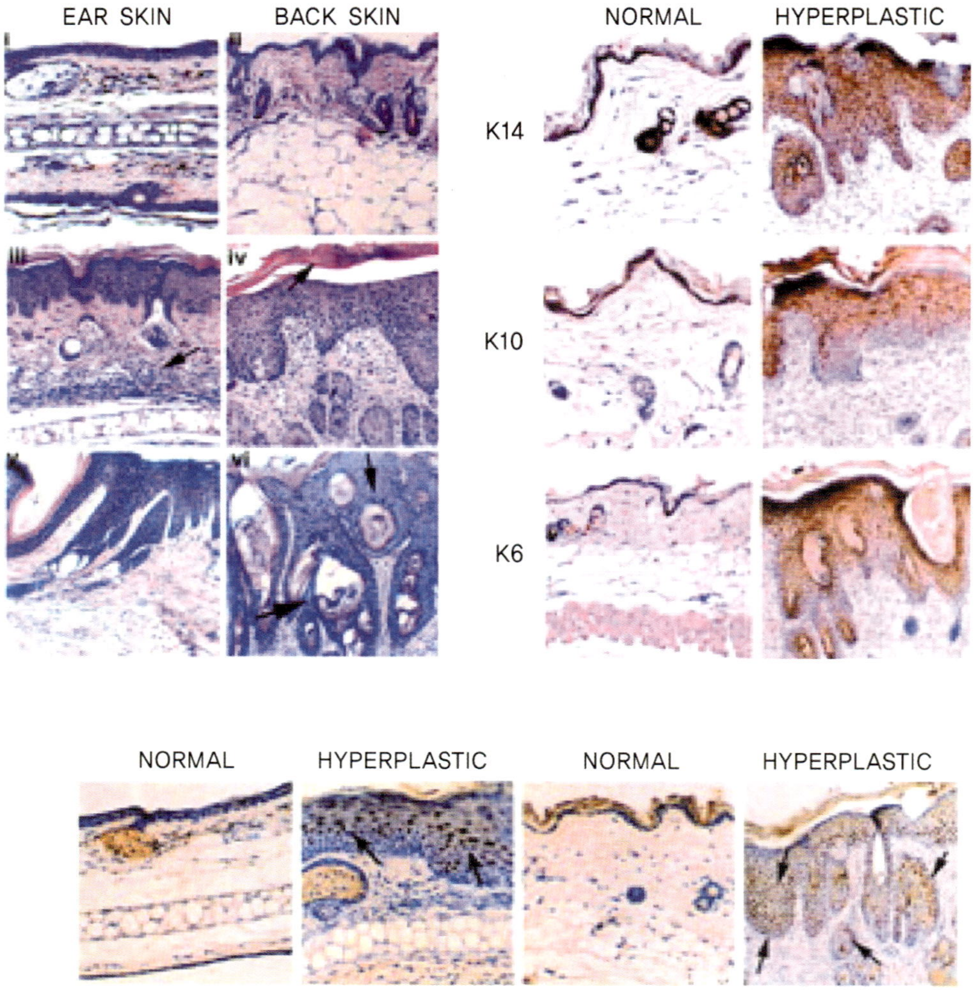

그림 14-5. Types of skin lesions–Secondary Lesions

dermis or corium : deeper layer (two layers ; connective tissue containing nerves, nerve endings, blood vessels, sebaceous glands(sebum=oil), and sweat glands (sudoriferous).

hair and nails : appendages of skin.

subcutaneous : under the skin ; contains adipose tissue, connective tissue, vessels, and nerves.

Ⅱ. Function of the system

1. Word root

actin/o	ray
adip/o, lip/o	fat
albin/o, alb/o, leuk/o	white
caus/o	burns
derm/o, dermat/o, cutane/o	skin
hidr/o	sweat
hydr/o	water
kerat/o, corn/i	horny, hard
leuk/o, albin/o, alb/o	white
lip/o, steat/o, stear/o	fat
melan/o	black
onych/o, ungu/o	nail
seb/o	sebum, sebaceum
squam/o	scale
syring/o	tube, fistula
top/o	place
trich/o, pil/o	hair
vesic/o	vesicle
xanth/o	yellow
xer/o	dry

2. Anatomical terms

dermis, corium	stratum corneum
epidermis	stratum germinativum
hair	stratum granulosum
papillary layer	stratum lucidum
reticular layer	stratum spinosum
sebaceous gland	sweat gland
sebum	

3. Medical terms

acne vulgaris : a chronic skin disorder usually occurring in adolescents and young adults, in which there is increased production of sebum from sebaceous glands and the formation comedones that plug the pores.

acne : a disorder of the skin with eruption of papules or pustules.

albinism : congenital abscence of normal pigmentation in the body(hair, skin, eyes).

allergic dermatitis : Familiar examples of the allergic type are poison ivy, oak, and sumac. These include rubber and plastics, industrial chemicals, cosmetics, clothing, dyes, costume jewelry, some animals and plants, detergents, insecticides and paints.

alopecia : loss of hair, baldness.

anesthesia : loss of feeling or sensation.

anhidrosis : abscence of sweating.

athlete's foot : a chronic superficial fungal infection of the skin of the foot, especially of that between the toe and on the sole.

bleb : a large flaccid vesicle, usually at least 1cm in diameter.

burn : injury to tissues caused by contact with dry heat(fire), moist heat(steam or liquid), chemicals, electricity, lightening, or radiation.

cellulitis : diffuse inflammation of the soft or connective tissue due to infection.

chloasma : hyperpigmentation in circumscribed areas of the skin; called also melasma.

cicatrix : the fibrous tissue left after the healing of a wound, scar.

comedo : a blackhead, a plug of keratin and sebum within the dilated orifice of a hair follicle frequently containing the bacteria.

common baldness : alopecia, especially absence of hair from the scalp.

contact dermatitis : there are two types ; allergic contact dermatitis and primary irritant dermatitis.

cosmetic operation : operation patient's appearence by plastic improved restoration, correction.

crust, scab : dried serum, blood or pus.

cutaneous candidiasis, moniliasis : it is ususlly a superficial infection of the moist cutaneous areas of the body.

dandruff : dry scaly material desquamated from the scalp.

debridement : the removal of necrotic tissue from adjacent to a infected lesion until surrounding healthy tissue is exposed.

decubitus ulcer : an ulcer due to local interference with the circulation; called also bedsore and pressure sore. The ulcer usually occurs over a bony prominence such as that of the sacrum, hip, heel, shoulder, or elbow.

dermabrasion : planing of the skin done by mechanical means.

dermatitis : inflammation of the skin. Dermatitis can result from various animal, vegetable, and chemical substances, from heat or cold, from mechanical irritation, from certain forms of malnutrition, or from infectious disease. The symptomas may include itching, redness, crustiness, blisters, watery discharges, fissures, or other changes in the normal condition of the skin.

dermatome : an instrument for cutting thin skin slices for skin grafts.

diascopy : examination with the diascope.

dry gangrene : dry gangrene occurs gradually and results from slow reduction of the blood flow in the arteries. There is no subsequent bacterial decomposition; the tissues become dry and shriveled. It occurs only in the extremities, and can occur with arteriosclerosis, in old age, or in advanced stages of diabetes mellitus. Buergers disease can also sometimes cause dry gangrene.

ecchymosis : a hemorrhagic spot, larger than a petechia, in the skin or mucous membrane, forming a nonelevated, rounded or irregular, blue or purplish patch.

eczema : a superficial inflammatory process involving primarily the epidermis.

epidermal cyst : an epithelial cyst of the skin.

epidermolysis bullosa : disease of the skin, marked by the development of bullae and vesicles.

erosion : loss of part or all of the epidermis.

erysipelas : a superficial cellulitis caused by Streptococci.

erythema : redness of the skin caused by congestion of the capillaries in the lower layers of the skin.

escharotomy : surgical incision through tight burn eschar.

exanthema : any cutaneous eruptive disease or fever.

excoriation : any superficial loss of substance, caused by scratching, rubbing.

folliculitis : inflammation of the follicle.

gangrene : the death of tissue, generally in considerable mass, usually associated with loss of vascular supply, and followed by bacterial invasion and putrefaction. The three major types of gangrene are moist, dry, and gas gangrene.

gas gangrene : gas gangrene occurs in wounds infected by anaerobic bacteria, among which are various species of clostridium, break down tissue by gas production and by toxins.

herpes : any inflammatory skin disease caused by a herpesvirus and characterized by the formation of small vesicles in clusters.

herpes simplex : an acute viral disease marked by groups of vesicles, each about 3 to 6mm in diameter, on the skin, often on the borders of the lips. It often accompanies fever, although there are other precipitating factors, such as the common cold, sunburn, skin abrasions, and emotional disturbances.

herpes zoster : an acute viral disease characterized by inflammation of spinal ganglia and by a vesicular eruption along the area of distribution of a sensory nerve, caused by the virus of chicken pox. The disease may appear in persons who have been exposed to chickenpox, and it sometimes accompanies other diseases such as pneumonia, tuberculosis, and lymphoma or is triggered by trauma.

homografts : a graft of tissue between individuals of the same species.

hydrotheraphy : remove the topical agent and clean the burned area.

hyperhidrosis : excessive perspiration due to overactivity of the sweat gland.

hyperkeratosis : hypertrophy of the horny layer of the skin.

hyperpigmentation : abnormally increased pigmentation.

hypertrichosis : excessive hair growth in areas usually not hairy.

hypopigmentation : a congenital or acquired decrease in melanin production.

ichthyosis : skin disorders due to hypertrophy of scaliness.

impetigo : infection of the skin characterized by grouped vesicles or pustules.

juvenile melanoma : a benign, pink to purplish red papule, usually on the face, especially cheeks, most commonly originating before puberty.

keloid : a sharply elevated, irregularly shaped, progressively enlarging scar, due to excessive collagen formation in the corium during connective tissue repair.

keratosis follicularis, darier's disease : itching crusting, verrucous papular growths.

keratosis pilaris : hyperkeratosis limited to the hair follicles.

leprosy : inflammatory disease caused by Mycobacterium leprae. It is a chronic communicable disease characterised by the production of granulomatous lesions of the skin, mucous membranes, peripheral nervous system. Called also Hansens disease.

leukoderma : an acquired condition with localized loss of pigmentation of the skin.

lichenification : thickening of the epidermis, with exaggeration of its normal markings so that striae form a criss-cross pattern, enclosing flat-topped, shiny, smooth quadrilateral facets between them.

macule : a stain, spot, or thickening; an area distinguishable by color or otherwise from its surroundings.

malignant melanoma : a malignant tumor, usually developing from a nevus and consisting of black masses of cells with a marked tendency to metastasis.

melanoderma : an abnormally increased amount of melanin in the skin due to either an increase in production of melanin by the melanocytes normally present or to an increase in the number of melanocytes, with production of hyperpigmented patches.

melanoma : any tumor composed of melanin-pigmented cells.

miliaria, prickly heat : a syndrome associated with sweat occuring in the skin.

moist gangrene : moist gangrene is caused by sudden stoppage of blood, resulting from burning by heat or acid, severe freezing, physical accident that destroys the tissue, a tourniquet that has been left on too long, or a clot or other embolism. At first, tissue affected by moist gangrene has the color of a bad bruise, is swollen, and often blistered.

necrolysis : separation of tissue due to necrosis.

panniculitis : inflammation of the panniculus apiposus.

papule : a small circumscribed, solid, elevated legion of the skin.

paronychia : an inflammation of the tissue surrounding the nail plate.

pediculosis : infestation with lice of the family pediculidae.

petechia : a minute, pinpoint, nonraised, perfectly round, purplish red spot caused by intradermal or submucous hemorrhage, which later turns blue or yellow.

porokeratosis : disease of the skin, usually of the hand and feets, characterized by hypertrophy of the horny layer about the ducts of the sweat glands.

psoriasis : a chronic, recurrent skin disease marked by discrete bright red macules, papules, or patches covered with lamellate silvery scales. The lesions appear most often on the scalp, knees, and elbows. It sometimes occurs in association with rheumatoid arthritis but the connection between the two disorders in not clear.

purpura : purplish or brownish red discoloration caused by hemorrhage into the tissues.

pustule : a small, elevated, circumscribed, pus-containing lesion of the skin.

pruritis : itching, It is common in many types of skin disorders, especially allergic inflammation and parasitic infestations.

pyoderma : a purulent infection of the skin.

rash, eruption : visible lesions of the skin due to disease, and marked by redness, prominence.

ringworm : a group of fungal disease of the skin of man and domestic animals caused by dermatophytes.

scales : heaped-up particles of horny epithelium.

scar, cicatrix : the result of hearing after destruction of some of the dermis.

skin carcinoma : malignant epithelioma of the skin.

skin ulcer : a local, superficial defect, or excavation, of the surface of tissue by the cellular necrosis.

solar keratosis : any horny growth, such as a wart or callosity, and is caused by excessive exposure to the sun.

steatoma, sebaceous cyst : a fatty mass retained within a sebaceous gland.

syphilis : a contagious venereal disease leading to many structural and cutaneous lesions.

syringoma : adenoma of sweat glands.

tinea : ringwarm ; a name applied to many different kinds of fungal infection of the skin.

tinea versicolor : a chronic, noninflammatory and usually symptomless disorder.

tingling : a pricklike thrill caused by striking a nerve.

urticaria : a vascular reaction of the skin marked by transient appearance of slightly elevated patches which are redder or paler than the surrounding skin and often attended by severe itching ; called also hives.

vesicle : a small circumscribed elevation of the epidermis containing a serous fluid ; a small blister.

warts, verruca : an epidermal tumor caused by a papilloma virus.

wheal : a localized area of edema on the body surface, often attended with severe itching and usually evanescent.

wood's light : ultraviolet radiation much used in the diagnosis fungus infection.

xeroderma : a dry, rough, discolored state of the skin.

Chapter
15 AUDITORY SYSTEM

I. Ears

external ear : auricle, or pinna, and ear canal.

middle ear : lined with mucous membrane ; three bones : malleus, incus, stapes.

inner ear : vestibule, semicircular canals, and cochlea.

tympanic membrane : ear drum or myringa ; separates middle ear from external ear.

cerumen : wax in ear canal.

eustachian tubes : from middle ear to pharynx(throat) ; equalize pressure.

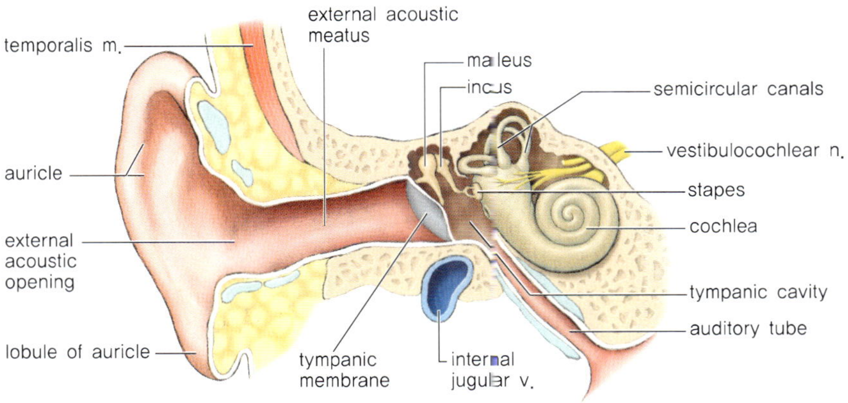

그림 15-1. Diagram of the ear showing outer ear canal, eardrum (tympanic membrane), middle ear, inner ear, and eustachian tube.

Ⅱ. Function of the system

1. Word root

aer/o	air, gas
audi/o, acous/o, acou/o	hearing
mastoid/o	mastoid process
meat/o	meatus
myring/o, tympan/o	eardrum, tympanic membrane
ot/o, aur/o, aur/i	ear
salping/o	eustachian tube
son/o, phon/o	sound

2. Anatomical terms

auricle	membranous labyrinth
cerumen	middle ear
cochlea	osseous labyrinth
endolymph	ossicle
external auditory meatus	oval window
external ear	perilymph
eustachian tube	round window
incus	semicircular canal
internal ear	stapes
labyrinth	tympanic cavity
malleus	tympanic membrane
mastoid process	vestibule

3. Medical terms

acoustic neuroma : benign tumor within the auditory canal arising from the acoustic nerve.

audiometer : an electronic device for the measurement of hearing.

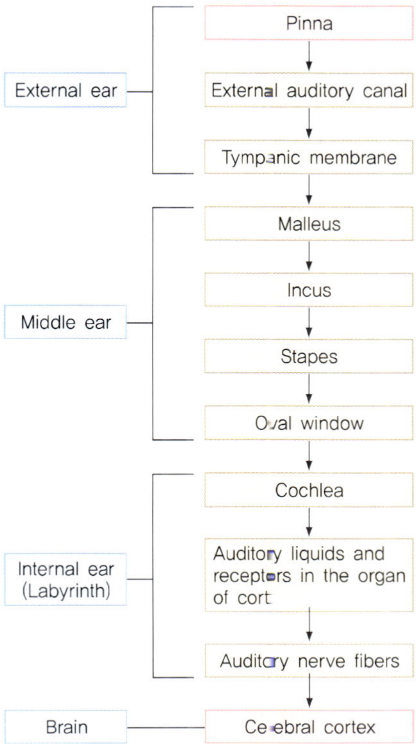

그림 15-2. Pathway of sound vibrations

audiometry : measurement of hearing, as by means of an audiometer.

aural atresia : absence or closure of the external auditory canal.

cerumen : a waxy secretion of the glands of the external acoustic meatus ; earwax.

cholesteatoma : a cystlike mass a lining of stratified squamous epithelium, filled with desquamating debris frequently including cholesterol, which occurs in the meninges, central nervous system, and bones of the skull, but most commonly in the middle ear and mastoid region.

chronic mastoiditis : an chronic inflammation of the mastoid antrum and cells.

deaf mutism : the absence both of the sence of hearing and of the faculty of speech.

deafness : lack or loss, complete or partial of the sense of hearing. The two major types of deafness are conductive deafness and sensorineural deafness. In conductive deafness sound vibration are interrupted in the outer or middle ear before they reach the nerve endings of the inner ear. In sensorineural deafness, the outer and middle ear function normmally, but damage to the nerve endings of the inner ear, the cochlear portion of the vestibulocochlear(eighth cranial) nerve, or the hearing center in the brain causes either interruption or confusion of the sound messages.

dizziness : a disturbed sense of relationship to space; a sensation of unsteadiness and a feeling of movement within the head, lightheadedness, disequilibrium.

ear speculum, otoscope : an instrument for exposing the interior of the ear.

eustachian curettage : the removal of growths or other material from the orifice of a eustachian tube, as with a curet.

eustachian salpingitis : inflammation of the auditory tube.

fenestration : the surgical creation of a new opening in the labyrinth of the ear for the restoration of hearing in otosclerosis.

hematotympanum : hemorrhagic exudation into the middle ear.

labyrinthitis : inflammation of the labyrinth ; otitis interna.

mastoidectomy : surgical removal of mastoid cells. The most frequent indication for mastoidectomy is chronic infection in the mastoid process occurring as a complication of chronic of diseased portions of the mastoid process as well as the incus and malleus of the middle ear and the tympanic membrane.

mastoiditis : inflammation of the mastoid antrum and cells. It is usually the result of an infection of the middle ear, with which the mastoid cells communicate. Mastoiditis most commonly follows sore throat and respiratory infection, but it can also fever. The symptoms include earache and a ringing in the ears.

menieres disease : a disorder of the labyrinth of the inner ear. It is believed to result from dilatation of the lymphatic channels in the cochlea. The usual symptoms are tinnitus heightened sensitivity to loud sounds, progressive loss of hearing, heacache and vertigo.

microtia : hypoplasia or aplasia of the pinna of the ear.

myringitis, tympanitis : inflammation of the tympanic membrane.

myringoplasty : surgical restoration of a perforated tympanic membrane by grafting.

myringorupture : forcible tearing of tympanic membrane.

myringotomy, tympanotomy : incision of the tympanic membrane.

nystagmus : involuntary, rapid, rhythmic movement of the eyes. Jerking nystagmus may be a sign of barbiturate intoxication, labyrin-thine-vestibular, vascular, or neurologic disease.

ossiculectomy : surgical removal of the ossicle of the ear.

otalgia : pain in the ear ; earache ; otocynia ; otoneuralgia.

othematoma : a collection of blood, usally clotted, in the ear.

otitis external : inflammation of the external ear.

otitis media : inflammation of the middle ear.

otoplasty : plastic surgery of the ear.

otorrhea : a discharge from the ear.

otosclerosis : the formation of spongy bone in the capsule of the labyrinth of the ear, often causing the auditory ossicles to become fixed and less able to pass on vibration when sound enters the ear.

otoscopy : examination of the ear by the otoscope.

petrositis : inflammation of the petrous portion of the temporal bone.

presbycusis, senile deafness : a progressive, bilaterally symmetrical perceptive hearing occuring with age.

salpingitis : inflammation of a uterine tube or the eustachian tube.

stapedectomy : excision of stapes.

tinnitus : a noise in the ears, as ringing, buzzing, or roaring, which may at times be heard by others than the patient.

vertigo : a sensation of rotation or movement of ones self or of ones surrounding in any plane. Vertigo may result from diseases of the inner ear or may be due to disturbances of the vestibular center or pathways in the central nervous system. The term is sometimes used erroneously as a synonym for dizziness.

Chapter 16

VISUAL SYSTEM

I. Eyes : rest in eye sockets ; orbital ridge of cranium(eyebrow area).

Parts of the eye

sclera : outer covering(rear part is the white of the eye ; clear front part is the cornea).

conjunctiva : mucous membrane covering of eye ; also lines eyelids.

choroid : dark-brown layer between sclera and retina(five layers) ; it is part of the uvea(iris, ciliary body, and choroid).

iris : colored band of choroid surrounding the pupil.

pupil : a hole in the iris ; the iris regulates the size of the pupil.

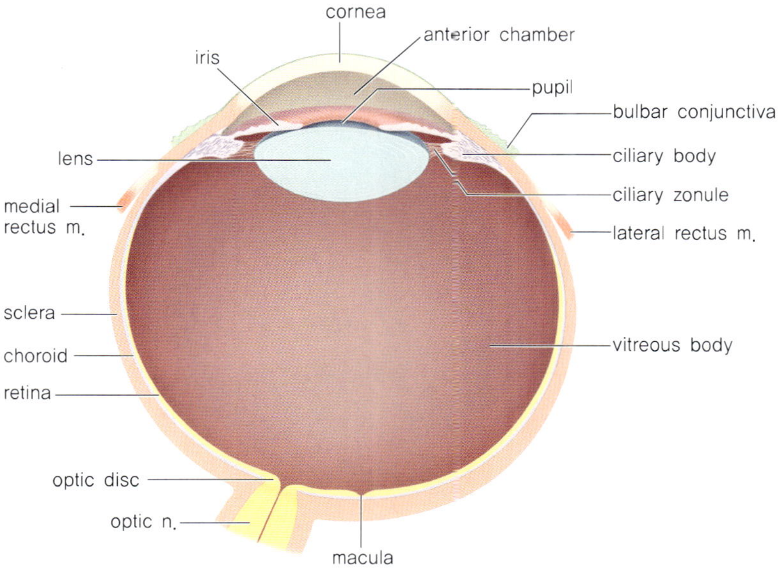

그림 16-1. Normal eye

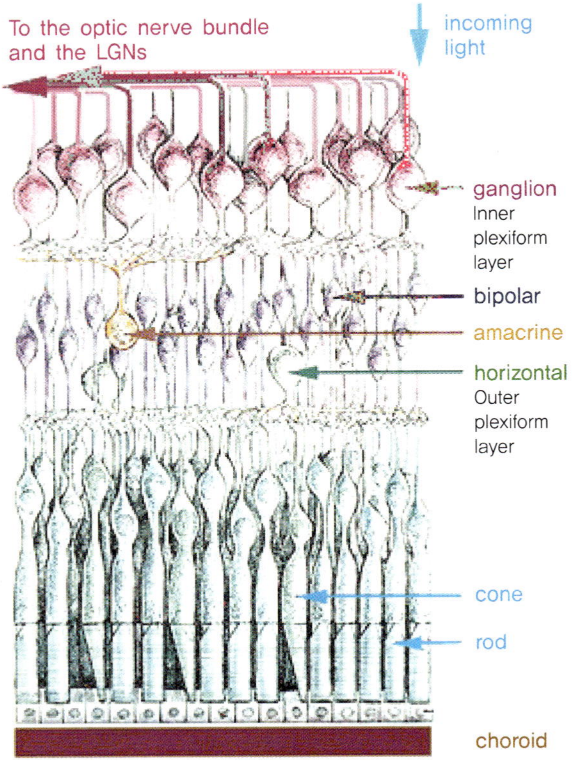

그림 16-2. Diagram of the microscopic structure of the retina

lens : transparent, colorless structure encapsulated and held in place behind the pupil by a ligament attached to the ciliary muscle.

aqueous humor : watery liquid in anterior chamber in front of the lens ; it circulates through the anterior and posterior chambers of the eye.

vitreous humor : jellylike transparent substance inside eyeball.

retina : innermost(third layer of the eye) that receives images formed by the lens ; contains sensitive nerve fibers ; connected with optic nerve. Muscles attached to the outside of the eyeball provide eye movements. The optic nerve transmits images to the brain. Lacrimal glands and ducts (tear glands) are located at the outer upper aspect of the eyes(called the lacrimal apparatus).

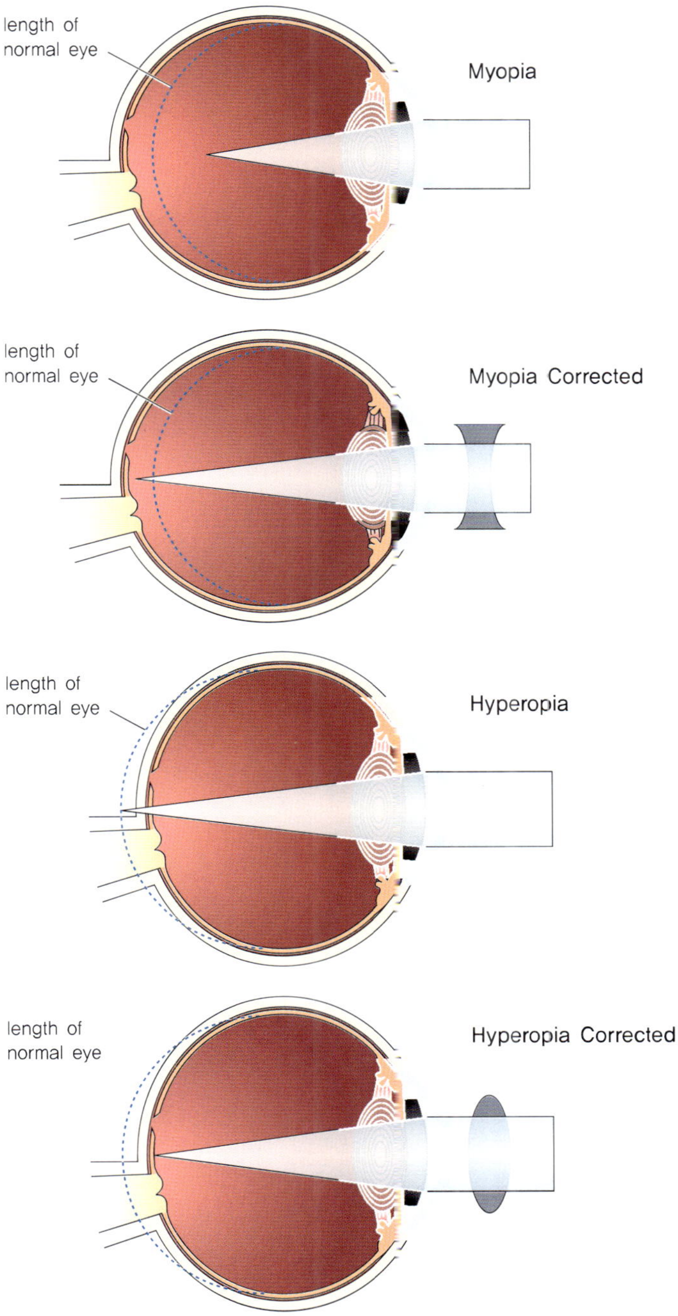

그림 16-3. Myopia and hyperopia

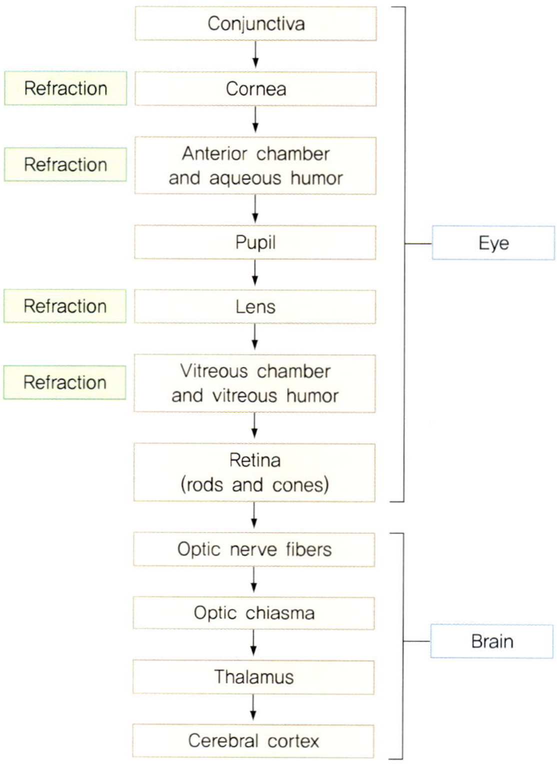

그림 16-4. Pathway of light rays

Ⅱ. Function of the system

1. Word root

blephar/o, palpebr/o	eyelid
corne/o, kerat/o	cornea
cycl/o	ciliary body of the eye
dacryocyst/o	lacrimal sac
dacry/o, lacrim/o	tears, lacrimal duct
ir/o, irid/o	iris
kerat/o, corne/o	cornea, horny tissue
lacrim/o, dacry/o	tear, lacrimal duct
opt/o	eye, vision
ophthalm/o, ocul/o	eye
phac/o, phak/o	crystalline lens
phot/o	light
presby/o	old age
pupill/o, cor/o	pupil
retin/o	retina
scler/o	sclera
tars/o	edge of the eyelid
typhl/o	blindness

2. Anatomical terms

anterior chamber	lacrimal duct
aqueous humor	lacrimal gland
blind spot	macula lutea
canthus	Meibomian gland
choroido	ptic disc or optic papilla
ciliary body	orbit
cilium	posterior chamber
conjuctiva	pupil
cornea	retina
crystalline lens	sclera
eyelid	tarsal plate
fovea centralis	uvea
iris	vitreous body

3. Medical terms

achromatopsia : the quality or the condition to being achromatic.

amaurosis : loss of sight without apparent lesion of the eye, as from disease of the optic nerve.

amblyopia : dimness of vision not due to organic defect or refractive errors.

amblyoscope : an instrument for training an amblyopic eye.

anisocoria : in aquality of the pupils in diameter.

astigmatism : an error of refraction in which a ray of light is not sharply focused on the retina, but is spread over a more or less diffuse area ; it is due to differences in curvature in various meridians of the refractive surfaces(cornea and lens) of the eye.

bepharoptosia : droping of an upper eyelid due to paralysis.

blepharitis : inflammation of the eyelids.

blepharophimosis : abnormal narrowness of the palpebral fissures in the horizontal direction.

blepharoplasty : plastic surgery of a eyelid.

blepharospasm : tonic spasm of the oribicularis oculi muscle, producing more or less complete closure of the eyelids.

blindness : lack or loss of ability to see.

blue sclera : a condition of unusual blueness of the sclera.

canthoplasty : plastic surgery of a canthus.

cataract : an abnormal progressive condition of the lens of the eye, characterized by loss of transparency. A graywhite opacity can be seen within the lens, behind the pupil.

cataract extraction : the surgical removal of a cataractous lens.

choroiditis : an inflammatory condition of the choroid membrane of eye.

chemosis : excessive edema of ocular conjuctiva.

chromop(s)ia : a visual defect in which colorless object appear to be tinged with color.

color sense test : examination about the distinction of various colors.

conjunctivitis : inflammation of the conjunctiva.

corneal laceration : tearing of the cornea.

cover-uncover test, cover test : a test for determining the type of phoria.

cryoextraction : the application of low temporature in the removal of a cataractous lens.

dacryoadenitis : inflammation of a lacrimal gland.

dacryocystectomy : excision of the wall of the lacrimal sac.

dacryocystitis : inflammation of the lacrimal sac.

dacryocystorhinostomy : a communication between the lacrimal sac and the nasal cavity.

diathermy : heating of the enucleated tissues, as the electromagnetic radiation, electric currents, or ultrasonic waves.

diplopia : the perception of two images of a single object.

ectropion : the turning outward of an margin of the eyelid.

enophthalmos : a backword displacement of the eyeball into the orbit.

epiphora : an abnormal overflow of tears down the cheek, mainly due to stricture of the lacrimal passages ; called also illacrmation.

exophthalmos : abnormal protrusion of the eyeball.

funduscopy : examination or inspection of the fundus of the eye.

glaucoma : an abnormal condition of elevated pressure within an eye owing to obstruction of the outflow of aqueous humor.

hordeolum, stye : a purulent inflammation of sebaceous glands of the eyelids.

hyperopia : a visual defect in which parallel light rays reaching the eye come to focus behind the retina, vision being better for distant objects than for near; called also hypermetropia and farsightedness.

hypertensive retinopathy : any noninflammatory disease of the retina associated with malignant hypertension.

iridectomy : surgical excision of part of the iris.

iritis : an inflammatory condition of the iris of the eye characterized by pain, lacrimination, photophobia, and if severe, diminished visual acuity.

keratitis : any inflammation of the cornea.

keratomalacia : softening of the cornea.

keratometer : an instrument for measuring the curves of the cornea.

keratoplasty, corneal graft : plastic surgery of the cornea.

keratotomy : surgical incision of the cornea.

leucoma cornea : a dense white opacity of the cornea.

light sense test : examination about the faculty distinguished the intensity of brilliancy.

macropsia : objects are seen as larger than they actually are.

maddox rods : a set of parallel cylindrical glass rods used in testing for heterophoria.

metamorphopsia : a disturbances of vision in which objects are seen as distorted in space.

micropsia : objects are seen as smaller than they actually are.

mydriasis : extreme dilatation of the pupil.

myopia : that error of refraction in which rays of light entering the eye paralled to the optic axis are brought to a focus in front of the retina, as a result of the eyeball being too long from front to back, so that vision for near objects is better than for far; called also nearsightedness and shortsightedness.

nyctalopia : night blindness.

nystagmograph : an instruments for recording the movements of the eyeball in nystagmus.

nystagmus : an involuntary rapid movement of the eyeball which may be horizontal, vertical, rotatory, or mixed.

ocular enucleation : removal of the eyeball.

ocular headache : pain in the head occuring around the eye.

ocular hypertension : persistently elevated intraoccular pressure.

ocular pain : pain in the eye.

ocular pro(s)thesis : an artificial substitute for the eyeball.

ophthalmitis : inflammation of the eye.

ophthalmodynamometry : determination of the retinal arterial pressure.

ophthalmoscopy : the examination of that interior of the eye with the ophthalmoscope.

optic neuritis : inflammation of the optic nerve.

orbital tumor : tumor occuring in the orbit.

papilledema : edema and hyperemia of the optic disk, usually associated with increased intracranial pressure; called also choked disk.

phorometer : an instrument for ascertaining the degree and kind of heterophoria.

photometer : a device for measuring the intensity of light.

photophobia : abnormal visual intolerance of light.

photopsia : an apearance as of sparks or flashes due to retinal irritation.

presbyopia, old sight : hyperopia and impairement of vision due to advancing years.

pupillometer : an instrument for measuring the width or diameter of the pupil.

redness, congestion : excessive or abnormal accumulation of blood in the eye.

reduced vision : loss of the act or facult of seeing.

refractive error test : measurement abcut the refractive error.

refractometer : an instrument for measuring the refractive power of the eye.

retinal detachment : a condition in which the retina are separated from the choroid.

retinitis : inflammation of the retina.

retinoblastoma : a malignant tumor arising from the retina.

retinopathy : any noninflammatory disease of the retina.

retinoscope : an instrument for evaluation and diagnosting refractive errors of the eyes.

scleral staphyloma : protrusion of the contents of the eyeball at a point where the sclera has become to thin.

scleritis : inflammation of the sclera.

sclerograft : transplant of the sclera.

strabismus : deviation of the eye that the patient cannot overcome; the visual axes assume a position relative to each other different from that required by the physiological conditions. Called also squint.

synechia : adhesion, as of the iris to the cornea or to the lens.

transilluminator : a device for the passage of light through the eye.

trichiasis : condition of ingrowing hairs about an orifice.

visual acuity test : measurement of clarity or clearness of the vision.

visual field test : examination about the portion of space which the fixed eye can see.

Chapter

17 ANESTHESIA TERMINOLOGY

I. Function of the system

1. Word root

aer/o	air
algesi/o	pain
bas/o	base
caud/o	tail
cephal/o	head
esthesi/o	feeling
hypn/o	sleep
narc/o	stupor

2. General terms

analeptics : stimulants of the central nervous system for example, coramine and caffeine.

analgesia : loss of normal sense of pain.

analgesics : drugs that relieve pain.

anesthesiologist : physician who specializes in anesthesiology.

anesthesiology : the science and study of anesthesia.

anesthetic : an agent producing insensibility to pain.

anesthetist : professional person, not necessarily a physician, who is qualified to administer anesthesia.

artificial ventilation : mechanism(respirator, ventilator) used to control rate and depth of breathing.

conduction anesthesia : term includes various forms of local anesthesia : direct, nerve block, epidural block, spinal anesthesia and infiltration anesthesia.

direct nerve block : in which anesthetic solution is injected into easily accessible nerves, as those in arms and legs.

endotracheal anesthesia : introduction of a catheter into the trachea in order to conduct the anesthetic mixture directly from the apparatus to the lungs. This may be achieved oral by or nasal intubation.

epidural block : spinal nerves are blocked as they pass through the epidural space.

field block : in which anesthetic solution in injected into the nerve at the point of its terminal branches.

hyperventilation : excessive respiration causing an abnormal loss of carbon dioxide from the blood.

hypoxia : a reduction of oxygen supply to body tissue.

infiltration anesthesia : dilute anesthetic agent is injected under skin to anesthetize the nerve endings and nerve fibers of that area.

inhalation anesthesia : general anesthesia produced by inhaling vaporized liquids or gases.

inhalation therapy : administration of inhalant gases such as oxygen, helium or carbon dioxide to relieve oxygen want to stimulate respiration.

intravenous anesthesia : IV administration of drugs to produce basal narcosis. A stage of unconsciousness is produced, but analgesia and muscular relaxation may prove unsatisfactory. Never used alone as an anesthetic.

lid reflex(LR) : tapping the eyelid to evoke its immediate closure. The lid reflex is a guide to determine the depth of anesthesia, since it is completely lost in a stage of anesthesia deep enough to permit major surgery.

malignant hyperthermia : an inherited, life-threatening syndrome usually characterized by a quick rise in body temperature, tachycardia, metabolic acidosis, increased creatine phosphokinase(CPK), and decreased calcium level. It may be initiated by potent anesthetic agents such as halothane or succinylcholine.

neuroleptanalgesics : potent anelgesics and tranquilizers producing detached quiescense and somnolence.

neuromuscular blocking agents, skeletal muscle relaxants : drugs that serve as adjuncts to general anesthesia by producing muscular relaxation and thus reducing the need for deep levels of anesthesia.

premedication : a combination of drugs including opium derivatives, barbiturates, belladonna and tranquilizers used in the preanesthetic preparation of the patient.

pudendal block : a nerve block affecting the external genitals, especially the female. Used extensively in obstetrics.

rectal anesthesia : rectal administraion of drugs to produce basal anesthesia.

sacral anesthesia : method of epidural anesthesia in which the anesthetic solution is injected into sacral canal.

spinal anesthesia : local anesthetic solution is injected into subarachnoid space of lumbar region to block roots of spinal nerves. Commonly used procaine HCL or xylocaine HCL.

surface or topical anesthesia : anesthetic drug is applied directly to mucous membrane or body surface in forms of location, ointment, or spray to produce insensibility of the nerve endings in the area. Cocaine HCL is useful surface anesthetic, as is xylocaine, procaine and novocain.

Chapter 18

MULTISYSTEM DISEASE

I. Function of the system

1. Word root

bacteri/o	bacterium
cac/o	bad, ill
immun/o	immune
myc/o, mycet/o	fungus, mycete
orrh/o, oro/o	serum
path/o	disease
-bacter	bacterium
-itis	inflammation
-pathy	disease

2. Congenital disorders

albinism : congenital absence of pigment in the skin, hair, and eyes, due to absence or defect of tyrosinase.

cystic fibrosis : systemic hereditary disease of unknown etiology seen in children and adolescents. It is characterized by a more or less extensive involvement of the exocrine glands, especially those secreting mucus and sweat.

down's syndrome : a congenital condition in which the afflicted child has mongoloid facies and senile features ; mental retardation usually occurs, which is mild to severe.

fabry's disease : a hereditary disease in which glycolipid are deposited in various tissues, especially the kidneys.

glycogen storage disease : a group of chronic, genetically determined metabolic disorders of childhood.

heredity : the genetic transmision of a particular quality or trait from parent to offspring.

klinefelter's syndrome : a gonadal abnormality caused by chromosomal aberrations and characterized by testicular dysgenesis, azoospermia, gyneomastia and mental deficiency.

mutation : a permanent transmissible change in the genetic materials, usually in a single gene.

neurofibromatosis : a familial condition characterized by developmental changes in the nervous system, muscles, bones, and skin.

turner's syndrome : gonadal abnormality affecting females caused by chromosomal aberration and characterized by amenorrhea, lack of breast development, dwarfism, mental deficiency and deafness.

3. Infectious diseases

actinomycosis : a fungal infection characterized by abscesses or granulomas of the cervicofacial lymph nodes, abdominal organs, and pulmonary tissues.

amebiasis : a protozoal infection which is affected the mucous membrane of the colon in the form of abscesses and ulcers. Abscesses may also occur in the liver, thoracic cavity, lungs, and skin.

ascariasis : found in the small intestine, causing pains and diarrhea, especially in children.

bacillary dysentery, shigellosis : acute infection caused by Shigella and marked by diarrhea, tenesmus, fever and in severe cases mucus bloody stool.

brucellosis, undulant fever : general infection by Brucella, characterized by intermittent or continuous fever, headache, chills, and profuse perspiration.

chancroid : a nonsyphilitic venereal disease transmitted by contact.

chicken pox, varicella : highly contagious infectious disease caused by the herpes zoster virus and characterized by sudden onset, mild fever, skin eruption.

clonorchis sinensis : the common liver fluke of man in China, Korea, Indochina, etc.

dermatophytosis : a fungous injection of the skin.

enterobiasis : pinworm infection usually found in children.

food poisoning : disease characterized by an abrupt onset of gastrointestinal symptoms caused by food intoxication or infection. Types are botulism, salmonellosis etc.

german measles, rubella : a mild viral infection characterized by a pink discrete and confluent macular exanthem.

gonorrhea : infection due to Neisseria gonorrhoeae transmitted venereally in most cases.

hookworm disease : infection by Necator americanus, which is attached to the intestinal mucosa.

leptospirosis : acute infection by one of the Leptospira species, transmitted to human beings by the ingestion of food that has been contaminated by the excretions of a reservior animal.

malaria : an infectious febrile disease caused by Protozoa.

measles, rubeola : highly contagious viral infection, clinically manifested by Kopliks spots of the buccal mucosa a rash, and catarrhal symptoms.

mumps : a contagious paramyxovirus disease, occuring mainly in children, characterized the inflammation and swelling of the parotids more so the submandibular or sublingual.

ornithosis : a contagious disease of nonpsittacine birds marked by respiratory and systemic infection.

rabies, hydrophobia : acute encephalitis that causes paralysis, delirium, convulsions, and death.

reye's syndrome : an acute, noncontagious viral illness of childhood that is characterized by encephalopathy and fatty hepatomegaly with brain swelling and central nervous system damage.

small pox, variola : an acute communicable viral infection characterized by an eruption of papules, followed by vesicles and pustules.

syphilis : a contagious venereal disease leading to many structural and cutaneous lesion, caused by the spirochete Treponema pallidum.

tuberculosis : diseases caused by Mycobacterium and characterized by the formation of tubercles and caseous necrosis in the tissues.

typhoid fever : a bacterial infection caused by a salmonella and characterized by gastrointestinal tract symptoms.

typhus : a rickettsial infection caused by a species of Rickettsia and transmitted by infected body lice, fleas, mites, ticks. Types are epidemic and murine forms.

4. Inflammatory diseases

inflammation : a localized protective response elicited by injury or destruction of tissues.

(1) Classification of inflammation

abscess : a localized collection of pus in a cavity formed by the disintegration of tissues.

acute inflammation : inflammation, usually of sudden onset

chronic inflammation : inflammation of slow progress.

fibrinous inflammation : inflammation that is characterized by an exudate of coagulated fibrin.

hemorrhagic inflammation : inflammation due to the hemorrhage.

pseudomembranous inflammation : inflammation characterized by the formation on a mucosal surface.

serous inflammation : inflammation which produces an exudation of serum.

subacute inflammation : a condition intermediate between chronic and acute inflammation.

suppurative or purulent inflammation : inflammation characterized by the formation of pus.

ulcer : a local defect, or excavation, of the surface of an organ or tissue.

(2) Systemic effect of inflammations

fever : elevation of body temperaure above the normal.

leukocytosis : a transient increase in the number of leukocytes in the blood.

leukopenia : reduction in the number of leukocytes in the blood.

5. Immunologic disease

acquired immune deficiency syndrome(AIDS) : concerted research efforts have not yet defined the actual causes of AIDS, although the infective agent is thought to be of viral origin and to be spread in bodily secretions, especially blood and semen.

amyloidosis : the accumulation of amyloid in various body tissues.

anaphylaxis : excessive hypersensitivity to foreign protein or other substance, clinically manifested by edema of the larynx, hypoxia, respiratory distress, hypotension and vascular collapse.

autoimmune disease : immunologic disorders in which the patients own tissues produce antigenic stimuli.

dermatomyositis : a nonsuppurative inflammation of the skin, subcutaneous tissue, and muscles.

hypersensitivity reaction : a state of a altered reactivity in which the body reacts with an exaggerated response to a foreign agent.

immune : being highly resistant to a disease.

immunological tolerance : an immunological response characterized by the develpment of specific nonreactivity of lymphoid tissues to a particular antigen.

polymyositis : inflammation of several or many muscles at once, along with degenerative and regenerative changes.

serum sickness : a hypersensitivity reaction following the administration of foreign serum and other antigens.

transplant rejection : hyperacute rejection reaction of an immune against grafted tissue.

transplantation immunity : immune responses to transplanting organs, depending on the histocompatibility of the type of graft.

Chapter 19 ONCOLOGY

Ⅰ. Function of the system

1. Word root

aden/o	gland
astr/o	star
carcin/o	carcinoma
epitheli/o	epithelium
lymph/o	lymph
onc/o	tumor
sarc/o	flesh
vas/o, angi/o	vessel, blood vessel
-carcinoma	carcinoma
-oma	tumor
-sarcoma	sarcoma

2. General terms

anatomic staging : the classification of neoplasms according to the extent of the tumor.

benign : not malignant ; not recurrent.

cancer : a cellular malignant tumor the natural course of which is fatal.

carcinoma : a malignant tumor made up of epithelial cells.

malignant : become progressively worse and to result in death.

metastasis : the transfer of disease from one organ or part to another directly connected with it.

radiosensitivity : sensitivity of the skin or other skin tissue to radiant energy.

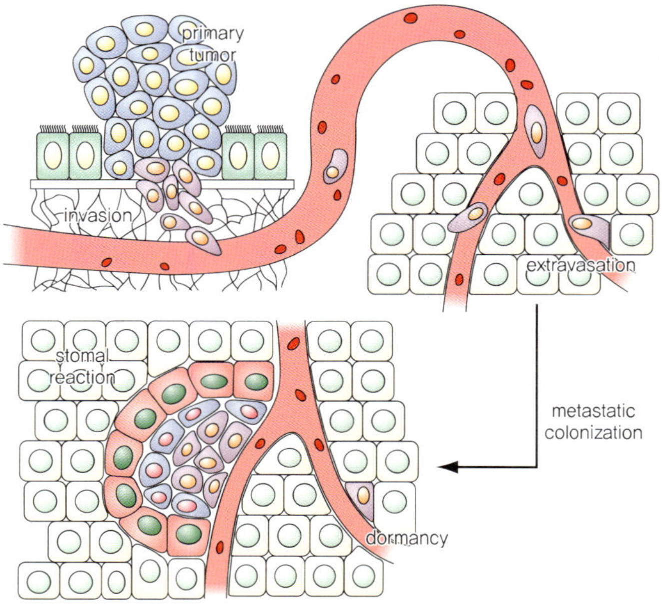

그림 19-1. Development type of tumor

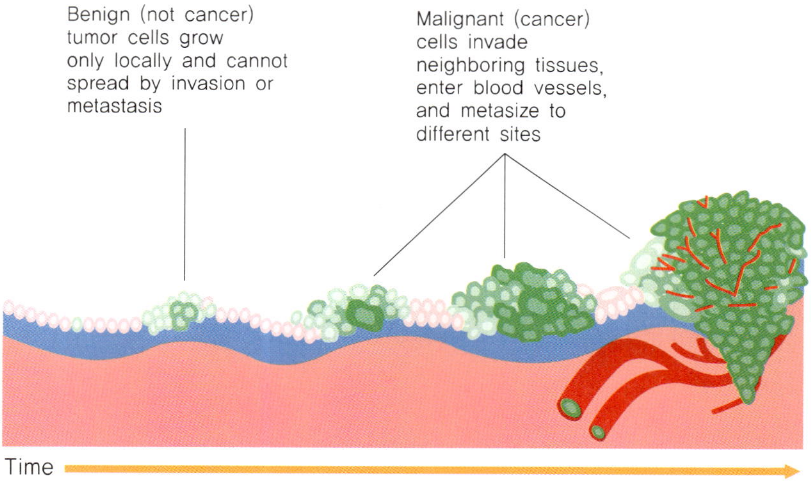

그림 19-2. Benign tumor and malignant tumor

sarcoma : a malignant tumor made up of a aubstance like the embryonic connective tissue.

TNM. staging TNM : staging of tumors according to three basic components ; primary tumor(T), regional lymphnodes(N), and metastasis(M).

ulcer : a local defect, or excavation, of the surface of tissue which is produced by the sloughing of inflammatory necrotic tissue.

3. Metastasis of tumors

pathways of spread(metastasis)

(1) **lymphatic, lymphogenous metastasis** : metastasis arising through the lymphatic vessel.

(2) **hematogenous metastasis** : metastasis from one tissue to another through the blood vessel.

(3) **disseminated, seeding metastasis** : when the malignant tumor penetrate into the natural open field of the body.

(4) **transplantation metastasis** : metastasis brought about by transfer of tumor cells by fluid and their implantation in a distant location.

4. Therapeutic and operative terms

(1) **Chemotherapy for cancer** : the treatment of cancer by chemical agents.

(2) **Immunotherapy** : treatment by the active immunity, passive immunity, immunopotentiatory and immunosuppressive.

(3) **Radiotherapy** : the treatment of disease by ionizing radiation.

(4) **Surgical operation** : any act performed with instruments or by the hands of a surgeon.

① **radical operation** : one involving extensive resection of tissue for the complete extirpation of disease.

excisional biopsy : biopsy of an entire lesion removed by excision.

incisional biopsy : biopsy of a selected portion of a lesion.

needle biopsy : biopsy of tissue by the punture of a tumor.

② specific surgical operation

cryosurgery : destruction of tissue by the extreme cold.

electrocoagulation : coagulation of tissue by means of a biterminal high frequency electric current.

laser peration : destruction of tissue by the laser.

5. Classification of tumors

(1) the anticipated behavior

(2) the histogenesis or cytogenesis

Histologic Derivation	Benign Neoplasms	Malignant Neoplasms	Site of Predilection
Connective tissue	Chondroma Lipona-benign neoplasm composed of adipose tissue(fat) Fiboma-benign mass or firm nodule of fibroblasts or fibrocytes Leiomyoma Rhabdomyoma-benign tumor arising in skeletal muscle	Sarcomas Chondrosarcoma Liposarcoma sarcoma composed of adipose tissue Fibrosarcoma Leiomyosarcoma malignant neoplasm of smooth muscle tissue Rhabdomyosarcoma-malignant, poorly differentiated, bizzare mass in striated muscle	Bones Fat Fibrous tissue Smooth(visceral) muscle Striated(skeletal) muscle
	Osteoid osteoma-benign tumor derived from osteoblastic tissue	Osteosarcoma, Osteogenic sarcoma	Long bones
Embryonal tissue	 Testicular adenoma	Choriocarcinoma Embryonal carcinoma of testis Seminoma	Uterus, testes, and mediastinum Testes Testes, epididymis, pelvic and paraaortic lymph nodes, and others

Histologic Derivation	Benign Neoplasms	Malignant Neoplasms	Site of Predilection
	Teratoma, mature-mixed tumor composed of any type of embyonic and adult tissue, as teeth, hair, bone, cartilage, and others.	Malignant teratoma, immature-mixed tumor malignant in one or the other tissue elements.	Testes,ovaries, and retroperitoneal and sacrococcygeal regions.
Epithelial tissue 1) Covering epithelium	Squamous cell papilloma	Carcinomas Epidermoid carcinoma Squamous cell carcinoma	Skin, buccal mucosa, tongue, salivary gland, lip, larynx, lung, blandder, anus, and others
		Oat cell carcinoma	Lung, esophagus and other sites of low incidence
		Basal cell carcinoma	Skin, especially face
2) Glandular epithelium	Adenoma	Adenocarcinoma	Breast, bronchi, digestive tract, pancreas, endocrine glands, prostate, and others
	Cystadenoma	Cystadenocarcinoma	Ovary, salivary gland, breast, and thyroid
	(a) serous type	(a) serous type-(rare)	Ovary
	(b) pseudomucinous type	(b) pseudomucinous type	Ovary
Hematopoietic or hematologic tissue		Leukemias	Blood

Oncology

Histologic Derivation	Benign Neoplasms	Malignant Neoplasms	Site of Predilection
Lymph-forming or lymphoid tissue		Lymphomas Hodgkin's lymphoma	Lymphocytes Lymphocytes
Nerve tissue or other tissue found in nervous system		Glioma group (a) Astrocytoma (b) Ependymoma (c) Glioblastoma multiforme (d) Oligodendroglioma Medulloblastoma Meningeal sarcoma	Brain Cerebellum Meningeal tissue
Nerve tissue	 Ganglioneuroma Neurilemoma-arising from periheral nerve Neurofibroma-tumor of peripheral nerve sheaths	Neuroblastoma Ganglioneuroblastoma Neurofibrosarcoma	Embryonic nerve tissue Mediastinum and retroperitoneum Nerve Nerve
Pigment forming tissue	Nevus	Malignant melanoma	Skin, eye, and extremities
Reticuloendothelial tissue		Ewing's sarcoma-malignant tumor of reticuloendothelial tissue Multiple myeloma, Plasma cell myeloma-malignant tumors derived from plasma cells of bone marrow	Bones Bones
Vascular tissue	Angioma Hemangioma-tumor of blood vessels Lymphangioma-tumor of the lymphatic vessels	Angiosarcona Hemangiosarcoma Lymphangiosarcoma	Blood vessel tissue Lymphatic vessels, neck, and others

Oncology

Chapter

20 PHARMACOLOGY

I. Function of the system

1. Word root

alg/o	pain
chem/o	chemistry, chemical
erg/o	work
idi/o	self, own
narc/o	stupor
pharmac/o	drug, medicine
pyr/o	heat, fire
tox/o, toxic/o	toxin, poison
vit/o	life
algesi-	pain
anti-, contra-	against, opposed
vita-	life
-phylaxis	protection against infection

2. Classification of drugs

(1) Drugs acting on the autonomic nervous system

parasympatholytic(cholinergic blocking) agent : an agent that opposes the effects of impulses conveyed by the parasympathetic nerves.

parasympathomimetic(cholinergic) stimulant : atropine.

sympathomimetic(adrenergic) agent : bronchodilator, vasoconstrictor, vasodilator

sympatholytic(adrenergic blocking) agent : propranolol(inderal).

(2) Drugs acting on the central nerve system

antipyretic analgesic : an agent that reduce fever and pain.

cerebral stimulant : an agent that produces stimulation of the central nervous system.

gerneral anesthetics : an agent that produces gerneral anesthesia. inhalation anesthesia, intravenous anesthesia, rectal anesthesia.

hypnotic : a drug that acts to induce sleep.

local anesthetics : an agent whose anesthetic action is limited to an area of the body. conduction anesthesia, infiltration anesthesia, spinal anesthesia, surface anesthesia.

muscle relaxant : an agent that aids in reducing muscle tension.

sedative : an agent that allays excitements.

vasoconstrictor : an agent that causes constriction of the blood vessels.

tranquilizer : drugs used in the treatment of anxiety states, neuroses and mental disorders.

(3) Drugs acting on the circulatory system

antihypertensive drug : an agent that reduces high blood pressure.

antilipemic agent : an agent that counteracts high levels of lipids in the blood.

cardiotonics : an agent that has a tonic effect on the heart.

coronary vasodilator : an agent that causes dilatation of the coronary artery.

migraine agent : an often familial symptom complex of periodic attacks of vascular headache.

(4) Drugs acting on blood and hematopoietic system

antianemic : an agent that counteracts or prevents anemia.

anticoagulant : an agent that prevent the coagulation of blood.

hemostatic : an agent that arrests the flow of blood.

(5) Drugs acting on the respiratory system

bronchodilator : an agent that causes expansion of the lung.

expectorant : an agent that promotes the ejection of mucous or exudate from the lungs, bronchi, and trachea.

(6) Gastrointestinal drugs

antacid : a substance that counteracts or neutralizes acidity, usually of the stomach.

antidiarrheal, obstipatic : an agent that is effective in combating diarrhea.

antiemetic : an agent that prevents nauses and vomiting.

cathartic : an agent that causes evacuation of the bowels.

cholagogue : an agent that stimulates the flow of bile into the duodenum.

digestant, digestive : an agent that or stimulates digestion.

emetic : an agent that causes vomiting.

stomachic : a medicine which promotes the functional activity of the stomach.

(7) Urogenital drugs

diuretic : an agent that promotes the excretion of urine.

oxytocic : an agent that hastens evacation of the uterus by stimulating contractions of the myometrium.

(8) The orthers

agent in diabetes mellitus : an agent usec in the treatment of the diabetes mellitus.

antibiotic : an agent that inhibit the growth of or kill other micro-organism.

anticancer agent : an agent that counteracts the effect of a cancer.

antihelmintic : an agent that is destructive to worms.

bactericide : an agent that destroys bacteria.

3. Administration of drugs

(1) Inhalation

(2) Injection : intracavitary injection
intradermal injection
intramuscular injection
intrathecal injection
intravenous injection
subcutaneous injection

(3) Oral administration

(4) Rectal administration

(5) Sublingual administration

Chapter

21 RADIOLOGY

I. Function of the system

1. Word root

electr/o	electricity
fluor/o	luminous
luc/o	light
radi/o	radiation
roentgen/o	x-ray
son/o, ech/o	sound
stere/o	three dimensions
therm/o	heat
tom/o	cutting
cine-	movement
tele-	far away
-gram	recorded
-graph	instrument for recording
-graphy	method of recording
-meter	instrument for measuring
-metry	method of measuring
-therapy	therapy

2. Introduction

body positions : body positions are the manner in which the patient is placed in relation to the surrounding space. The following terms are used to describe body positions:

erect position
oblique position
recumbent position
dorsal recumbent position(supine)
ventral recumbent position(prone)
lateral recumbent position(lying on side)
sitting position

contrast media : a radiopaque substances used to facilitate roentgen visualization of internal structures of the body.

method : some radiologic procedures are named after individuals(for example, Chassard Lapine or Towne) in recognition of their having developed a method to demonstrate a specific anatomic part. The method describes the position of the body in reference to established anatomic landmarks. In addition, the method describes the position of the film and central ray in relation to the body position.

projection : projection is the process of recording a body part on an image receptor(film). Projection usually describes the path of radiation as it goes from the x-ray tube through the patient to the image receptor.

radiation : electromagnetic waves, such as those of light, or particles rays, such as alpha, beta, and gamma rays, given off from some source.

radiography : film records of internal structure of the body by passage of X ray or gamma rays through the body.

radiology : the science of radiant energy and radiant substances, especially that branch of the health sciences which deals with the use of radiant energy in the diagnosis and treatment of disease.

1) diagnostic radiology : x-rays are used in a variety of ways to detect pathological conditions.

2) nuclear medicine : medical speciality that studies the characteristics and uses of radioactive substances in the diagnosis and treatment of disease.

3) radiation therapy(radiotherapy) : treatment of disease using an external source of high energy X-rays and gamma rays or internally implanted radioactive substances.

view : view describes the representation of an image as seen from the vantage of the image receptor. In comparing the definitions of view and projection, it must be noted that they are exact opposites. For many years view and projection were often used interchangeably, which led to confusion.

3. General terms

abdominal aortography : roentgenography of arteries after injection of contrast medium into the abdomanal aorta.

amniocentesis : surgical transabdominal perforation of the uterus, to obtain amniotic fluid.

angiocardiography : roentgenography of the heart and great vessels after introduction of contrast medium into a blood vessel.

aortography : radiography of the aorta after the intravascular injection of contrasrt medium.

arthrocentesis : puncture and aspiration of a joint.

bronchography : radiography of the bronchus after the injection of contrast medium into the bronchus.

cerebral angiography : radiography of the vascular system of the brain after injection of contrast medium into the artery.

chest radiography : a projection of the thoracic viscera shows the lungs, trachea, aorta, pulmonary regions.

coronary arteriography : roentgenography of arteries after injection of contrast medium into the coronary artery

dacryocystography : radiographic demonstration of dacryocyst and the nasolacrimal duct after injection of the contrast medium into the dacryocyst.

diskography : radiography of the spine for visualization of an inter-vertabral disk after injection of the contrast medium into a disk.

hysterosalpingography : radiography of the uterus and uterine tubes after the injection of contrast medium through the vagina.

knee arthrography : radiography of knee joint after injection of contrast medium into the patellofemoral joint.

laryngography : radiography of the larynx after the injection of contrast medium into the larynx.

lumbar puncture : the tapping of the subarachnoid space in the lumbar region.

lymphangiography : roentgengraphy of the lymphatic vessels following the injection of contrast medium.

myelography : radiography of the spinal cord after injection of contrast medium into the subarachnoid space.

nuclear medicine : in vivo(counting) study(tyroid scan, brain scan, liver scan), in vitro study.

operative cholangiography : cholangiography performed during a surgical procedure on the gallbladder.

pelvimetry : the measurement of the dimensions and capacity of the pelvis.

placentography : radiological visualization of the placenta after the injection of a contrast medium.

pneumoarthrography : radiographic of a joint after the injection of air or gas.

pneumoencephalography : radiographic visualization of the fluid containing structures of the brain after the injection of air or gas.

pneumoventriculography : radiography of the cerebral, ventricules after the injection of air or gas.

prostatography : the detection of calcareous deposits and as shown by urinary retention, of prostatic enlargement.

radiation therapy : brachytherapy, curative irradiation, fixed field technique, palliative irradiation, rotation therapy technique, teletherapy.

retrograde pyelography : radiography of the kidney, ureter and bladder in which the contrast medium is injected into the renal pelvis through the urethra.

retrograde urethrography : radiography of the urethra after the injection of an contrast medium through the urethra.

sialography : radiographic demonstration of salivary ducts by means of the injection of contrast medium.

thoracocentesis : surgical punture of the chest wall into the parietal cavity for aspiration of fluids.

ventriculography : radiography of the head after injection of contrast medium into the cerebral ventricles.

voiding cystourethrography : radiography of the urinary bladder and urethra in which the radiography made before, during and after voiding.

xeroradiography(soft tissue X-ray) : a dry, totally photoelectric process for recording X-ray image, using metal plates coated with a semiconductor.

Chapter

22 ABBREVIATIONS

General hints regarding abbreviations

Periods are generally omitted. Some abbreviations are shown in capital letters ; some will be seen in either capitals or lower case letters.

AP anterior/posterior

D disease

F Fellow

L/R left/right

N national

P physicians

S surgeons, syndrome

U/L upper/lower

GENERAL ABBREVIATIONS

A anterior, accommodation, atrium, artery

AA Alcoholics Anomymous, Associate of Arts (degree)

aa of each (pharmacy)

AAA abdominal aortic aneurysm

AAE active assistive exercise (physical therapy)

A & D admission and discharge (hospital department)

A & P (or P & A) auscultation and percussion (listening and tapping)

A & P repair anterior/posterior repair of perineum

A & W alive and well

AAR acute anxiety reaction

AAT alpha 1-antitrypsin ; used in deficiency related emphysema

ab abortion (if spontaneous, same as miscarriage)

ABC airway breathing circulation

ABG arterial blood gases aspiration biopsy cytology

ABO Landsteiner blood groups

ABS acute brain syndrome

ac before meals

AC air conduction

ACTA type of scanner

ACTH adrenocorticotropin hormone

AD right ear(auris dextra)

ADC Aid to Dependent Children (also AFDC, families)

ADH antidiuretic hormone

ADHD Attention deficit hyperactivity disorder

ADL activities of daily living

ad lib as desired, at will

ADR Adriamycin (antieoplastic drug)

AE above elbow (amputation)

AFB acid-fast bacillus (TB and related organisms)

AGA approximate gestational age (length of pregnancy)

$AgNO_3$ silver nitrate (instilled in newborns eyes to prevent GC)

AI artificial insemination

AIDS acquired immune deficiency syndrome

AJ ankle jerk (reflex)

AK above knee (amputation)

AL axillary line (right or left)

ALL acute lymphocytic leukemia

ALP alkaline phosphatase (high in Ca of prostate)

ALS amyotrophic lateral sclerosis (Lou Gehrig's disease), antilymphocyte serum

AMD actinomycin D (antineoplastic drug)

AMI acute myocardial infarction

AML acute myeloblastic (myelocytic, myelogenous)leukemia

ANA antinuclear antibodies (lab test ; presence may indicate autoimmune disease), American Nurse's Association

ANLL acute nonlymphocytic leukemia

ANS autonomic nervous system

AP anterior/posterior

APC aspirin, phenacetin, caffeine (analgesic medication)

APGAR score of newborns condition (Dr. Apgar)

APL anterior/posterior/lateral

Aq aqueous (water)

ARA C(Ara C) cytosine arabinoside(antineoplastic drug)

ARC AIDS related complex

ARDS acute (adult) respiratory distress syndrome

ARE active resistive exercise

ART Accredited Records Technician

AS left ear (auris sinistra), aortic stenosis

ASA acetylsalicylic acid (aspirin)

ASAP as soon as possible

ASCVD arteriosclerotic and cardiovascular (orcerebrovascular)disease

ASD atrial septal defect (congenital heart defect)

ASHD arteriosclerotic heart disease, atirial septal heart defect

as tol as tolerated (diet, and so on)

Au gold(metallic element; salts used in treatment; radioactive gold used in certain Ca cases and liver scan)

AV arteriovenous (shunt), atrioventricular

AVR aortic valve replacement

AZT Aschhein-Zondek test (for pregnancy), drug used in treatment of

AIDS(zidovudine)

B bacillus, buccal

B_6 pyridoxine vitamin

Ba barium (opaque substance used in x-ray procedures)

B/A backache

Bab Babinski reflex (neurologic test ; normal in infant but abnormal after 6 months)

BaE barium enema (also BE)

baso basophil (white blood cell type)

BBB bundle branch block (heart) ; L or R ; blood brain barrier

BBT basal body temperature

BCG Calmette-Guerin (TB bacillus) used as vaccine

BCP blood chemistry profile

BD birthdate

BE barium enema, below elbow(amputation)

BEAM brain electrical activity mapping in diagnosis of tumors, epilepsy

BEB benign essential blepharospasm

BHA bilateral (or benign) hilar adenopathy

BID, bid twice a day

BK below knee

BM bowel movement

BMR basal metabolic rate

BMT bone marrow transplant

BOW bag of waters(amniotic sac)

BP(B/P) blood pressure

BPH benign prostatic hypertrophy

BRP bathroom privileges

BS bowel sounds, breath sounds, blood sugar

BSA body surface area (important measurement in burn patients)

BSP bromosulphthalein (lab)

BT bleeding time, brain tumor, body temperature

BU Bodansky units(lab term)

BUN blood urea nitrogen (lab test of kidney function)

BVR Bureau of Vocational Rehabilitation

BW birth weight, body weight

Bx biopsy

C centigrade, celsius, costal(rib), cervical, carbon, cesarean

c cubic, centimeter

$\bar{c}$ with

C-1, C-2, and so onncervical first, second, and so on vertebra or spinal nerve

CA cancer, carcinoma, chronologic age

Ca calcium, cancer

CABG cabbage (coronary artery bypass graft)

CAD coronary artery disease

cal calorie

C & S culture and sensitivity (bacteriology lab)

caps capsules

CAT computerized axial tomography (also CT)(scan) ; multiple x-rays fed into computer provide cross sections of multiple planes

cath catheterized

CBC complete blood count

CBD common bile duct, closed bladder drainage

CBS chronic brain syndrome

CC chief or current complaint, crippled children, compensation case ; cardiac catheterization

cc cubic centimeter (also written cm^3)

CCI chronic coronary insufficiency

CCU coronary care unit

CD communicable disease

CDA certified dental assistant

CDC Centers for Disease Control, communicable disease center

CF Christmas factor (in blood, bleeding disorder), cystic fibrosis, complement fixation

CHD coronary heart disease, congenital heart disease

CHF congestive heart failure

CHO carbohydrate

CLL chronic lymphocytic leukemia

cm centimeter (cm3=cubic centimeter), costal margin (left or right)

CML chronic myelocytic leukemia

CMV cytomegalo virus

CN cranial nerve (also written Cr I, Cr II, and so on)

CNS central nervous system

Co cobalt (chemical element, used in Ca treatment)

CO carbon monoxide

CO_2 carbon dioxide

COLD see COPD

comp compensation

COPD chronic obstructive pulmonary disease (also COLD, chronic obstructive lung disease)

CP cerebral palsy

CPD cephalopelvic disproportion (in birth canal, head too large)

CPK creatinine phosphokinase (enzyme released when heart or muscle is damaged)

CPM cyclophosphamide (antineoplastic drug)

CPR cardiopulmonary resuscitation

CPT current procedural terminology(codes)

CPZ chloropromazine (drug)

CRF chronic renal failure, corticotro-pin releasing factor

crit hematocrit (blood test)

CRP(A) C-reactive protein (antiserum)

CS central service(supply), coronary sinus

C section cesarean section (caesarean)

CSF cerebrospinal fluid

CSR central supply room

CT see CAT

Cu copper (metal) ; small quantities used by body

cu cubic

cu cm cubic centimeter(cm^3)

cu mm cubic millimeter(mm^3)

CV cardiovascular, cerebrovascular

CVA cerebrovascular accident (stroke) ; cardiovascular accidentcva

cva costovertebral angle (area over the kidney)

CVD cardiovascular (carebrovascular) disease

CVP central venous pressure; Cytoxan, vincristine, prednisone (combination of drugs used in cancer treatment)

CVS chorionic villus sampling of placenta (for fetal defects)

CW crutch walking

CXR chest x-ray (procedure)

cysto cystoscopy

D dorsal, diopter, disease, divorced

d deceased, dead, distal, dorsal

D & C dilatation and curettage (uterus)

D & D diagnosis and dispostion

D-1, D-2, and so onndorsal (thoracic) vertebra spinal, nerve, or rib

DAT diet as tolerated

db decibel (unit of sound)

DC(D/C) discontinue, discharged, Doctor of Chiropractic

DD differential diagnosis, dry dressing

DDP Division of Disease Prevention

DDS Doctor of Dental Surgery

DDT insecticide

DES diethylstilbestro(hormone)

DHS Department of Health Services

DI diagnostic imaging ; diabetes insipidus

DIC disseminated intravascular clotting

diff differential (count of each type of WBC)

DIP distal interphalangeal (joint)-joint near tip of finger

DJD degenerative joint disease

DK diet kitchen

DLE disseminated lupus erythematosus

DM diastolic murmur, diabetes mellitus

DMD Doctor of Medical Dentistry

DMSO dimethyl sulfoxide (controversial drug)

DNA deoxyribonucleic acid (present in chromosomes of nuclei cells, carries genetic information)

DNR dorsal nerve root

DNS did not show(for appointment)

D/ns (D/s) dextrose in normal saline(IV solution)

DO Doctor of Osteopathy or Optometry

DOA dead on arrival

DOB date of birth

dorsi dorsiflexion (of foot, turned to posterior aspect of body as in pointing toes)
DOU definitive observation unit (just below intensive care)
DPT diphtheria, tetanus, pertussis (immunization) ; also DTP, DT
DR dorsal root, doctor, dressing
DRG diagnostic related groupings
DSD dry sterile dressing
DTP same as DPT
DTR deep tendon reflex
DTs delirium tremens (in alcoholism)
DVR Department of Vocational Rehabilitation
DVT deep vein thrombosis
D/W dextrose in water (DW=distilled water)
Dx diagnosis

E enema, eye, extremity
EA educational age
E & H environment and heredity
EBV Epstein Barr virus
ECF extended care facility ; extracellular fluid
ECG electrocardiogram
ECHO virus (enterocytopathogenic human orphan virus)
echo sound
ECM erythema chronicum migrans(skin lesion in Lyme disease)
E. coli Escherichia coli(bacterium)
ECT electroconvulsive therapy (shock treatment)
ED emergency department
EDC estimated date of confinement (due date for delivery)
EEG electroencephalogram (brain wave recording)

EFP(R) effective filtration pressure (rate)

EGD esophagogastroduodenoscopy

EIA/ELISA enzyme immunosorbent assay or enzyme linked immunosorbent assay. Screening tests on blood samples to detect presence of HIV antibodies

EKG electrocardiogram

EM electron microscope

EMG electromyogram (muscle)

EMI type of scanner

EMT emergency medical technician

ENG electronystagmography (to test vestibular function by assessing eye motion)

ENT ear, nose, and throat

EOM extraocular movements

eos, eosin eosinophil(type of white blood cell)

ER emergency room, external rotation

ERCP endoscopic retrograde cholangiopancreatography

ERT estrogen replacement therapy

ERV expiratory residual volume (pulmonary function test)

ES emergency service

ESP extrasensory perception

ESR erythrocyte sedimentation rate(blood test)

EST electroshock therapy (same as ECT)

ETOH ethynol, ethyl alcohol

EUA examination under anesthesia

ext external

F Fahrenheit, female, Fellow, frequency

FACP, FACS Fellow of American College of Physicians, Surgeons

FANA fluorescent antinuclear antibodies

FAS fetal alcohol syndrome

FB, Fb fingerbreadth, foreign body

FBS fasting blood sugar

FDA Food and Drug Administration

Fe iron

$FeSO_4$ ferrous sulfate

FEV forced expiratory volume

FF force fluids

FH family history

FHT fetal heart tones

F-N finger to nose(coordination)

FOB fiberoptic bronchoscopy, foot of bed

FP flat plate(x-ray procedure)

Fr French(catheter)

FROM full range of motion (of joint)

FS frozen section

FSH follicle-stimulating hormone

FTA fluorescent treponemal antibody (syphilis test)

FTND full-term normal delivery

FU;5-FU fluorouracil(cancer drug)

FUO fever of undetermined origin

Fx fracture

G glucose, gingival, specific gravity

g(Gm, gm) gram(unit of weight) ; 29 g in 1 oz

Ga gallium (rare metal, used in scans)

GA gestational age, gastric analysis

GAS general adaptation syndrome, group A streptococcal infection

GB gallbladder

GBS gallbladder series (x-ray film)

GC gonorrhea (sexually transmitted disease)

GE gastroenteritis

GFR glomerular filtration rate (kidney test)

GG gamma globulin (protein in blood, used therapeutically for passive temporary immunity)

GH growth hormone

GI, GIS gastrointestinal, series (x-ray film)

GP general practitioner, gram positive

gr grain, gravida, gravity

gram cystogram (x-ray film of bladder), unit of weight

Grav Ⅰ,Ⅱ, and so onngravida Ⅰ, Ⅱ, and so on(number of pregnancies)

GT, GTT glucose tolerance(test)

gtt drop

GU genitourinary

GV gentian violet(dye used in lab and as topical medication)

GVHD graft versus host disease

gyn gynecology

H hydrogen, hypo

H^+ hydrogen ion

h hour

H_2O water

Hb, Hgb hemoglobin (iron containing pigment in BCs, carries oxygen to tissues)

HBO hyperbaric oxygen therapy

HBP high blood pressure (hypertension)

HCl hydrochloric acid (normal in the stomach)

HCO_3 bicarbonate

Hct hematocrit (blood test, low in anemias)

HCTZ hydrochlorothiazide (diuretic)

HD Hodgkins disease (type of cancer), Hansens disease (leprosy), hip disarticulation ; Huntingtons disease

HDL high-density lipoprotein (good cholesterol)

HEENT head, eyes, ears, nose, throat

HEW Health, Education, and Welfare ; see HHS

HF high frequency (sounds)

Hg mercury (metallic element)

Hgb hemoglobin

HGH human growth hormone

HH hard of hearing

HHS Health and Human Services

HID headache, insomnia, depression (syndrome)

HIV human immunodeficiency virus

HLA homologous (human) leukocytic antibodies

HMD hyaline membrane disease (of newborn babies)

HMO Health Maintenance Organization

HNP herniated nucleus pulposus (hemnia of intervertebral disc)

h/o history of

HOH hard of hearing

HP high power field (microscope) ; hemipelvectomy

HS heart sounds, head sling

hs bedtime

HSG hysterosalpingography(gram)

HSO hysterosalpingooophorectomy

HSV herpes simplex virus(causes cold sores, genital herpes)

HTLV human T-lymphotropic virus type Ⅲ

HVD hypertensive vascular disease
hypo injection, hypoglycemic diet
Hx history

I iodine (nonmetallic element, used as medication and in diagnosis of thyroid disorders)
^{131}**I** radioactive isotope of iodine
I & D incision and drainage
I & O intake and output
IBS irritable bowel syndrome
IC intensive care, intercostal
ICA internal carotid artery
ICD International Classification of Diseases
ICF intracellular fluid
ICM intercostal margin
ICN intensive care nursery
ICP intracranial pressure
ICS intercostal space
ICT insulin coma therapy
ICU intensive care unit
IDDM insulin dependent diabetes mellitus
IgA immunoglobulin A
IH infectious hepatitis
IHD ischemic heart disease
IHSS idiopathic hypertrophic subaortic stenosis
IM intramuscular (injection)
IND investigational new drug
INH isoniazid (TB drug)
in situ in position or original place (not metastasized)

IOP intraocular pressure

IPPB intermittent positive pressure breathing (treatment)

IQ intelligence quotient

ITP idiopathic thrombocytopenic purpura

IU international units

IUD intrauterine device(for contraception)

IV intravenous (into vein)

IVC intravenous cholangiogram, inferior vena cava

IVD intervertebral disk (bewtwen vertebrae)

IVDA IV drug abuser

IVDU IV drug user

IVF in vitro fertilization

IVP intravenous pyelogram (x-ray film of kidney)

J joint, journal, Jewish

K potassium (mineral) essential in diet

KAB knowledge, attitudes and beliefs (or behaviors) survey

KCl potassium chloride (one of the ingredients in Ringers solution for IV)

KD knee disarticulation

kg kilogram

KJ knee jerk(reflex)

$KMnO_4$ potassium permanganate (antiseptic)

KRP Kolmer Reiter protein (syphilis test)

KS Kaposis sarcoma

KUB kidneys, ureters, bladder

KVO keep vein open (do not allow IV to run dry)

L liter, left, lower, lumbar

L-1, L-2 and so onnfirst, second, and so on lumbar vertebra or spinal nerve

L I, L II, L III primary, secondary, tertiary lues(syphilis)

LA left atrium or auricle (of heart)

L & A light and accommodation (eye)

L & D labor and delivery

L & W living and well

LASER light amplification by stimulated emission of radiation (has some uses in surgery)

lat lateral

LATS long acting thyroid stimulator

Lav lymphadenopathy associated virus

LCM left costal margin

LD Lyme disease

LDH lactic dehydrogenase (enzyme, lab test)

LDL low density lipoproteins (bad cholesterol)

LE lupus erythematosus, lower extremity, left eye

LGI lower gastrointestinal (series), same as barium enema

LH luteinizing hormone

LKS/np liver, kidney, spleen (also LSK-liver, spleen, kidney) nonpalpable

LLB lower leg brace

LLL lower left lobe, lower left lid

LLQ lower left quadrant

LMP last menstrual period (to calculate due date)

LN lymph node

LOA, LOP left occiput anterior, posterior (presentation at delivery)

LOC loss of consciousness

LOM limitation of motion

LP lumbar puncture, low power(microscope)

LPN licensed practical nurse(LVN-licensed vocational nurse)

LRQ lower right quadrant

LRS lactated Ringers solution (for IV)

LS lumbosacral

LSD d-lysergic acid (hallucinogenic drug)

LTB laryngotracheobronchitis (croup)

LTH luteotropic hormone (pituitary hormone, prolactin)

LUL left upper lobe

LUQ left upper quadrant

LV left ventricle

LVH left ventricular hypertrophy

lymph lymphocyte (type of blood cell)

M mean, medium, male, married, medical, morphine, murmur, mortality, morbidity

M_1 first mitral sound, heart sound at apex

m murmur, minim, monocyte, meter

MA mental age, menstrual age, Master of Arts, mentum anterior (presentation at delivery)

M & M morbidity and mortality

MAO monoamine oxidase (inhibitor) (type of medication)

MAST medical antishock trousers

mcg microgram

MCH mean corpuscular hemoglobin (blood test), maternal and child health

MCHC mean corpuscular hemoglobin concentration (Hgb in each RBC or per unit of blood)

MCV mean corpuscular volume (measurement of size of individual red cell)

MD Doctor of Medicine, muscular dystrophy

MEG magnetic encephalography

mEq/L milliequivalent per liter (measurement of concentration of a solution)

MF meat free(diet)

MFD minimal fatal dose

MG myasthenia gravis

mg(mgm) milligram

MH mental health, marital history

MI myocardial infarction, mitral insufficiency

mL(ml) milliliter(same as cc)

MM mucous membrane

mm millimeter

mm^3 cubic millimeter

mmHg millimeters of mercury

MMPI Minnesota Multiphasic Personality Inventory (test)

MMR measles, mumps, rubella (combined immunization)

MMWR Morbidity and Mortality Weekly Report(by CDC)

MO mineral oil

MOM Milk of Magnesia mono mononucleosis, monocyte (white blood cell)

MOPP nitrogen mustard, Oncovin, prednisone, procarbazine (drugs used in combination for some cancers)

MOR minor operating room

MR may repeat, metabolic rate, mentally retarded, medical records

MRI magnetic resonance imaging (scanner and computer)

MRL medical records librarian

MS multiple sclerosis, mitral stenosis, morphine sulfate, muscle strength, musculoskeletal

MT medical technologist(lab)

MT(ASCP) medical technologist (American Society of Clinical Pathologists)

MTX methotrexate(cancer drug)

MVA motor vehicle accident
MVP mitral valve prolapse(heart valve)
MVR mitral valve replacement

N nitrogen, negative, normal, national
n normal(saline), nasal, nerve
NI, NII, and so onnnerves by number
N_2O nitrous oxide(anesthetic gas)
Na sodium
NaCl sodium chloride(salt)
NAD no acute distress
$NaHCO_3$ sodium bicarbonate
n & t nose and throat
n & v nausea and vomiting
NB newborn
NBM nothing by mouth
NED no evidence of disease
NER no evidence of recurrence
NFTD normal full term delivery
NG nasogastric(tube)
NGU, NSU nongonorrheal urethritis, nonspecific urethritis
NH_3 ammonia
NIDDM noninsulin dependent diabetes mellitus
NIH National institute of Health
nm neuromuscular
NMR nuclear magnetic resonance (gives chemistry cf an organ)
NP neuropsychiatric, nasopharygeal
NPH neutral protein Hagedorn (insulin)
NPN nonprotein nitrogen(lab test)

NPO nothing by mouth, nothing per os

nr no repeat(no refill ox Rx)

ns normal saline(salt solution equal in concentration to that of body fluids)

NSAID nonsteroid antiinflammotory drug(pronounced en-sed)

NYD not yet diagnosed

O occiput, oculus, oral, oxygen

O_2 oxygen

OA occiput anterior, old age, osteoarthritis

OAA old age assistance

O & C onset and course

OASI old age and survivor's insurance

OB obstetrics

OB-GYN obstetrics-gynecology

OBS organic brain syndrome

OC oral contraceptive

OCG oral cholangiogram(bile ducts x-ray film)

OD right eye, overdosed, Doctor of Optometry, occupational disease

od every day ; once a day

OHS open heart surgery

OI opportunistic infection

OIDS Office of Infectious Disease Services

OJ orange juice

OOB out of bed

OPD outpatient department

OR operating room

ORIF open reduction internal fixation

ORT operating room technician

OS left eye

OSHA Occupational Safety and Health Administration

OT occupational therapy

OTC over the counter(medications)

OTR occupational therapist registered

OU both eyes, each eye

OV office visit

P phosphorus, pulse, passive, proximal, pupil, para (live births)

p post, pupil(of eye), para, p wave(ECG)

PA posterior/anterior, pulmonary artery, pernicious anemia

PABA para-aminobenzoic acid(sunscreen preparation)

PAD peripheral arterial disease

PAN periarteritis nodosa

P & A percussion and auscultation (tapping and listening)

PaO_2 arterial oxygen pressure

PAP primary atypical pneumonia

Pap Papanicolaou(smear for cancer detection)

Para Ⅰ, Ⅱ, and so onnnumber of live births, full term

PAT paroxysmal atrial tachycardia

PBI protein bound iodine(thyroid test)

PBZ pyribenzamine(antihistamine medication)

pc after meals

PCA patient controlled analgesia

pcn, PCN penicillin

pCO_2 pressure of tension of carbon dioxide

PCP pneumocystis carinii pneumonia

PCV packed cell volume

PD Doctor of Pharmacy

Abbreviations

PDA patent ductus arteriosus(open duct between pulmonary artery and aorta)

PDR Physician's Desk Reference(listings of prescription drugs)

PE physical examination ; pulmonary embolism

Peds pediatrics

PEEP positive endexpiratory pressure

PEG pneumoencephalogram

PELA percutaneous excimer laser angioplasty

PERRLA pupils equal, round, react to light and accommodation (eye)

PF push fluids

pg pregnant

PGH pituitary growth hormone

pH hydrogen ion concentration (measure of acidity/alkalinity)

PH past history, public health

PICA posterior inferior cerebellar artery

PID pelvic inflammatory disease

PIIS posterior inferior iliac spine

PIP proximal interphalangeal joint

PKU phenylketonuria(causes retardation)

PM physical medicine, postmortem, afternoon

PMI point of maximum intensity

PMN polymorphonuclear(leukocyte)

PMS premenstrual syndrome

PN peripheral nerve, practical nurse

PND paroxysmal noctural dyspnea, postnasal drip

PNS peripheral nervous system

PO phone order, postoperative, per os(orally)

PO_2, pO_2 pressure of oxygen

PO_4 phosphate(important in acid-base balance of blood)

POD postoperative day

POMP prednisone, Oncovin, methotrexate, 6-mercaptopurine(combination of cancer drugs)
PP postprandial(after a meal)
PPD purified protein derivative(TB test), permanent partial disability
PPH primary pulmonary hypertension
PPLO pleuropneumonia-like organism(causes atypical pneumonia)
PRE progressive resistive exercise
prn as needed
PROM premature rupture of membranes
PSP phenolsulfonphthalein(renal excretion test)
PSRO professional standards review organization
PT physical therapy, prothrombin time
pt patient
PTA prior to admission
PTCA percutaneous transluminal coronaryangioplasty (compression of atherosclerotic plaque to increase diameter of lumen)
PTD permanent total disability
PTH parathyroid hormone
PUD peptic ulcer disease
PVC/B premature ventricular contractions/beats
PVD peripheral vascular disease
pvO_2 venous oxygen pressure
PWA person with AIDS
Px prognosis
PZA pyrazinamide(TB drug)
PZI protamine zinc insulin

q every
QA quality assurance

qd every day

qh, q2h every hour, every 2 hours

qid four times a day

qm every morning

qn every night

qns quantity not sufficient(for test ordered)

qod every other day

QRS complex(ventricular complex in ECG)

qs quantity sufficient

R, r right, rectally, resistant, roentgen, respiration

Ra radium

RA rheumatoid arthritis, right atrium, residual air

RAD, rad radiation absorbed dose (unit of measure for x-rays)

RAI radioactive iodine

RAIU radioactive iodine uptake

RATx radiation therapy

RBC red blood cell, red blood count

RBD right border dullness

RBF renal blood flow

RC Red Cross, respiratory center, red cell, Roman catheter

RCD relative cardiac dullness

RCM right costal margin

RD retinal detachment(eye), respiratory disease

RDS respiratory distress syndrome

RE right eye, readmission

REM rapid eye movements(during dreams)

rep repeat

RF respiratory failure, rheumatic fever, rheumatoid factor

Rh factor in blood(Rh$^+$ have thefactor)

RHD rheumatic heart disease

RhoGAM injection given to Rh-negative women after delivery, miscarriage, or abortion to prevent antibody formation against Rh factor

RLF retrolental fibroplasia(eye condition that causes blindness)

RLL right lower lobe

RLQ right lower quadrant

RML right middle lobe, right mediolateral(episiotomy)

RMSF Rocky Mountain spotted fever

RNA ribonucleic acid

R/O rule out

ROA right occiput anterior (presentation at delivery)

ROAD reversible obstructive airway disease

ROM range of motion, rupture of membranes

Rom Romberg(neurologic test for balance)

ROP right occiput posterior(presentation)

ROS review of systems

RP retrograde pyelogram

RPR rapid plasma reagent(syphilis test)

RPT registered physical therapist

RRA Registered Records Administrator

RRL Registered Records Librarian

RRT Registered Respiratory Therapist

RSB right sternal border

RSV respiratory syncytial virus

RT radiotherapy, recreational therapy, radiologic technologist

RTC return to clinic

RUE right upper extremity

RUL right upper lobe

RUQ right upper quadrant
RV right ventricle, residual volume, rubella virus
RVH right ventricle hypertrophy
RVHD rheumatic valvular heart disease
Rx prescription, recipe, treatment, therapy
rx reaction

S, s sacral, stimulus, sulfur, sinister (left), saline, sensitive, section
$\overline{\text{s}}$ without
S-1 first sacral spinal nerve or vertebra
SA sinoatrial node(pacemaker in heart), sarcoma
SAD seasonal affective disorder (lack of light)
SAH subarachnoid hemorrhage
SB stillborn, sternal border (right/left, upper/lower)
SBE subacute bacterial endocarditis
Sc subcutaneously
SC sickle cell
SCUBA self-contained underwater breathing apparatus
SD shoulder disarticulation
sed sedimentation rate(rate at which blood settles)
seg segmented white blood cells (mature forms with segmented nuclei)
SF salt free
sg, sp, gr specific gravity(weight as compared to water)
SGOT serum glutamic oxaloacetic transaminase(enzyme, lab test)
SGPT serum glutamic pyruvic transaminase(enzyme, lab test)
SH serum hepatitis(hepatitis B), social history
SHS Sayre head sling
SIADH syndrome of inappropriate antidiuretic hormone
S/ICU surgery/intensive care unit

SIDS sudden infant death syndrome

sig let it be labeled (label on prescription)

SIJ sacroiliac joint

SLB short leg brace

SLC short leg cast

SLE systematic lupus erythematosus(LE)

SMA, SMAC 6, 12 or 18 sequential multiple analysis (series of blood chemistry tests)

SMR submucous resection(nasal surgery)

SNAFU situation normal, all fouled up

SNDO standard nomenclature of diseases and operations

SO_4 sulfate

SOB short of breath

SOL space occupying lesion

soln solution

SOPM stitches out in afternoon

sp gr specific gravity

sq, subq subcutaneously

Sr strontium(metallic element)

SR sedimentation rate, systems, review, sinus rhythm, stimulus/response

SS social service, Social Security, soap solution, sterile solution, saline soak, supersaturated, signs and symptoms

ss one half

SSE soapsuds enema

SSKI saturated solution potassium iodide(medication)

stabs nonsegmented white blood cells(immature forms)

staph Staphylococcus(bacterium)

stat immediately

STD sexually transmitted disease, skin test dose

STH somatotropin(growth hormone)

strep Streptococcus(bacterium)

STS serologic test for syphilis

subq, subcu subcutaneously

SV stroke volume

SVC superior vena cava

SW short wave(diathermy)

Sx signs, symptoms

T, t temperature, thoracic, total, tetanus, tablespoon

T-1, T-2, and so onnfirst, second, and so on thoracic vertebra or spinal nerve

T+1, T+2 increased intraocular tension

T-1, T-2 decreased intraocular tension

T_3, T_4 thyroid function tests

TAB typhoid, paratyphoid A and B(vaccine), therapeutic abortion

tab tablet

TAH total abdominal hysterectomy

T & A tonsillectomy and adenoidectomy, tonsils and adenoids

T & C turn and cough

T & R treated and released

TAT toxin antitoxin, toxoid antitoxin, tetanus antitoxin, Thematic Apperception Test

Tb, Tbc tubercle bacillus, tuberculosis

TBW total body weight

TC tissue culture

TCDB turn cough deep breaths

TCNS transcutaneous electrical nerve stimulation(also TENS, TNS)

TED thromboembolus(support hose to prevent emboli)

temp temperature, temporal
TENS transcutaneous electrical nerve stimulation
TF tuning fork
TH thyroid hormone
THA total hip arthroplasty
THI thiamine
THR total hip replacement
TIA transient ischemic attack
tid three times a day
tinc, tr tincture(alcohol preparation)
tiw three times a week
TKA total knee arthroplasty
TKO to keep open(vein)
TKR total knee replacement
TL tubal ligation(sterilization)
TLA translumbar aortogram
TLC total lung capacity, tender loving care
TLCA transluminal coronary angioplasty
TM tympanic membrane, temporomandibular
TMJ temporomandibular joint(jaw)
TNC too numerous to count(lab)
TNM tumor, nodes, metastasis (cancer staging system)
TNS transcutaneous nerve stimulation
TO telephone order
TOF tetralogy of Fallot(congenital heart defect)
TP total protein, testosterone pro-prionate, Treponema pallidum
TPA tissue plasminogen activator
TPC Treponema pallidum complement test(syphilis test)
TPI Treponema pallidum immobilization test

TPN total parenteral nutrition

TPR temperature, pulse, and respirations

TPUR transperineal urethral resection

Tr trace, tincture, traction

trach trachea, tracheotomy, tracheostomy

TSB total serum bilirubin(lab test)

TSH thyroid stimulating hormone

TSS toxic shock syndrome

TT tilt table, transfer to

TTD temporary total disability, transverse thoracic diameter

TTH thyrotropic hormone

TUR, TURP transurethral resection of prostate gland

TV tidal volume, total volume, television

TVC timed vital capacity (pulmonary function test)

TW tap water

Tx traction, treatment, tumor cannot be assessed

U unit, upper, uranium

UA(or Ua) urinalysis

U & C urethral and cervical

UC uterine contractions

UCG ultrasound cardiogram

UE upper extremity(arm)

UG urogenital

UGI upper Gi series(x-ray film)

ULQ upper left quadrant

UN urea nitrogen(lab test) ; same as BUN

ung ointment

UNOS United Network Organ Sharing

U/O under observation
UR Utilization Review
URI upper respiratory infection
URQ upper right quadrant
U/S ultrasound
USP US Pharmacopoeia(list of medications)
USPHS US Public Health Service
UTI urinary tract infection
UV ultraviolet

V ventricle, volt, volume, virulence, valve, vein, Roman numeral for number 5
VA Veterans Administration, visual acuity
VC vital capacity, vocal cord
VCG vector cardiogram
VCR vincristine(cancer drug)
VCU voiding cystourethrogram
VD venereal disease
VDRL Venereal Disease Research Laboratories
Vf ventricular fibrillation, visual field
VR vocational rehabilitation, venous return, ventral root
VS vital signs
VSD ventricular septal defect
VZ virus varicella-zoster(shingles)

W water, week, wesk, widow, with, watt, weight, width, wife
WAIS Wechsler Adult Intelligence Scale
WB whole blood
WBC white blood count, white blood cell
WBC & diff white blood count and differential(count of each type WBC)

WC wheelchair

WD well developed, wet dressing

WDWN well developed, well nourished

W/F, wf white female

WHO World Health Organization

WISC Wechsler Intelligence Scale for Children

W/M, wm white male

WN well nourished

WNL within normal limits

WP wet pack, whirlpool

WPW Wolff-Parkinson-White syndrome(disturbance in conduction in Purkinje fibers of heart)

X cross(match), cross section, Roman numeral for 10

X ray roentgen ray

XU excretory urogram

XX female chromosome

XY male chromosome

Y/O year old

Z zero

Zn zinc

SYMBOLS

♂ male

♀ female

〉 greater than

〈 less than

± plus or minus

↑ increased, elevated

↓ decreased, lowered

// parallel

→ to the right

← to the left

↔ stable unchanging

✔ check

number, divide

≠ not equal to

Physical therapy abbreviations

Kinds of Treatment

E. stim electrical stimulation

fluido fluidotherapy

FTx Fontaine traction

HP hot pack

HT Hubbard tank

IC Tx intermittent cervical traction

IP Tx intermittent pelvic traction

MWD microwave diathermy

parr paraffin(wax)

PT physical therapy

STx Sayre traction

SWD shortwave diathermy

TENS transcutaneous electrical nerve stimulation

US ultrasound

WP whirlpool

WT wading tank

Movement

AAROM active assistive range of motion

abd abduction

add adduction

AROM active range of motion

elev elevation

ER external rotation

ext extension

flex flexion

IR internal rotation

lat flex lateral flexion

PROM passive range of motion

ROM range of motion

SAQ short arc quad

SLR straight leg raise

General

act. active

act assist active assistive

ADL activities of daily living

AE amp above elbow amputee

a g antigravity

AK amp above knee amputee

amp amputation

BE amp below elbow amputee

BIW twice a week

BK amp below knee amputation

FOB foot of bed

ft foot or feet

FWB full weight bearing
LLE left lower extremity
LUE left upper extremity
MED minimal erythemal dosage
NWb non weight bearing
II bars parallel bars
pass passive
PRE progressive resistive exercise
pt patient
PWB partial weight bearing
reed reeducation
rehab rehabilitation
RLE right lower extremity
RUE right upper extremity
Rx treatment or therapy
SB side bending
TIW three times a week
TO telephone order
Tx traction
WC wheelchair
W / cm^2 watts per centimeter squared
WFL within functional limits
wt weight
x times or repetitions

Pulmonary function abbreviations

CaO_2 concentration of oxygen in arterial blood
CcO_2 concentration of oxygen in end capillary blood
$C\bar{v}O_2$ concentration of oxygen in mixed venous blood

DL_{CO} diffusing capacity of the lung for carbon monoxide
DLO_2 diffusing capacity of the lung for oxygen
ERV expiratory reserve volume
$FECO_2$ fraction of carbon dioxide in expired air
$FEF_{25\%\sim75\%}$ forced midexpiratory flow(between 25% and 75% of FVC)
FEN_2 fraction of nitrogen in expired air
FEO_2 fraction of oxygen in expired air
FEV_1 forced expiratory volume in 1 second
FEV_3 forced expiratory volume in first 3 seconds
FIN_2 fraction of nitrogen in inspired air
FIO_2 fraction of oxygen in inspired air
FRC functional residual capacity
FVC forced vital capacity
IC inspiratory capacity
IRV inspiratory reserve volume
MVV maximum voluntary ventilation
$P\bar{A}_{CO}$ mean partial pressure of carbon monoxide in alveolar gas
$PACO_2$ partial pressure of carbon dioxide in alveolar gas
$P\bar{A}CO_2$ mean partial pressure of carbon dioxide in alveolar gas
$PaCO_2$ partial pressure of carbon dioxide in arterial blood
P_{alv} alveolar pressure
PAH_2O partial pressure of water in alveolar gas
Pao pressure at airway opening
PaO_2 partial pressure of oxygen in arterial blood
PA_{O_2} partial pressure of oxygen in alveolar gas
$P\bar{A}O_2$ mean partial pressure of oxygen in alveolar gas
PB atmospheric pressure
Pbs pressure at external surface of chest
PCO_2 partial pressure of carbon dioxide

$P\bar{c}O_2$ mean partial pressure of oxygen in capillary blood
$P\bar{E}CO_2$ mean partial pressure of carbon dioxide in mixed expired air
P_t recoil pressure of lung
pN_2 partial pressure of nitrogen
PO_2 partial pressure of oxygen
Ppl pleural pressure
PRS recoil pressure of total respiratory system
PW recoil pressure of chest wall
$\dot{Q}t$ total cardiac output
$\dot{Q}x$ shunt flow
R respiratory exchange ratio
Raw resistance of tracheobronchial tree to flow of air into lung
Re Reynolds number
RQ respiratory quotient
RUS resistance of upstream segment of tracheobronchial tree
RV residual volume
Sao_2 percentage saturation of hemoglobin with oxygen in arterial blood
SO_2 percentage saturation of hemoglobin with oxygen
TLC total lung capacity
$\dot{V}$ gas volume per minute
V_1 inspiratory volume of ventilation per minute
VA volume of alveolar gas
$\dot{V}A/\dot{Q}c$ ratio of alveolar ventilation to pulmonary blood flood
Vc volume of blood in pulmonary capillary bed
VC vital capacity
$\dot{V}_{CO}$ rate of carbon monoxide uptake per minute
$\dot{V}CO_2$ amount of carbon dioxide eliminated per minute
VD volume of dead space gas
$\dot{V}E$ expiratory volume of ventilation per minute

$\dot{V}_{max}$ maximal rate of airflow during forced expiration

$\dot{V}_{max50}$ rate of airflow at 50% of vital capacity

$\dot{V}_{O2}$ rate of oxygen uptake per minute (oxygen consumption)

VT tidal volume(also TV)

Cancer abbreviations

This list is presented to acquaint the student with some abbreviations used in cancer cases. The breast is used as an example for the anatomic site of cancer ; however, terms dealing with tumor size are generally applicable.

Primary Tumor(T)

TX tumor cannot be assessed

TO no evidence of primary tumor

TIS Pagets disease of the nipple with no demonstrable tumor

T1 tumor 2 cm or less in greatest dimension

$T1_a$ no fixation to underlying pectoral fascia or muscle

$T1_b$ fixation tu underlying pectoral fascia and/or muscle

Ⅰ tumor-0.5 cm or less

Ⅱ tumor-more than 0.5~1.0 cm or less

Ⅲ tumor-more than 1.0~2.0 cm or less

T2 tumor more than 2 cm but not more than 5 cm in greatest dimension

$T2_a$ no fixation to underlying pectoral fascia or muscle

$T2_b$ fixation to underlying pectoral fascia and/or muscle

T3 tumor more than 5 cm in its greatest dimension

$T3_a$ no fixation to underlying pectoral fascia or muscle

$T3_b$ fixation to underlying pectoral fascia and/or muscle

T4 tumor of any size with direct extension to chest wall or skin(chest wall includes ribs, intercostal muscles, and serratus anterior muscle, but not pectoral muscle)

T4$_a$ fixation to chest wall

T4$_b$ edema(including peau d'orange), ulceration of the skin of the breast, or satellite skin nodules confined to the same breast

T4$_c$ both of the above

Lymph nodes(N) (definitions for clinical diagnostic stage)

NX regional lymph nodes cannot be assessed clinically

N0 homolateral axillary lymph nodes not considered to contain growth

N1 movable homolateral axillary nodes considered to contain growth

N2 homolateral axillary nodes considered to contain growth and fixed to one another or to other structures

N3 homolateral supraclavicular or infraclavicular nodes considered to contain growth, or edema of the arm(edema of the arm may be caused by lymphatic obstruction, and lymph nodes may not then be palpable)

Lymph nodes(N) (definitions for surgical evaluative and postsurgical treatment pathologic)

NX regional lymph nodes cannot be assessed(not removed for study, or previously removed)

N0 no evidence of homolateral axillary lymph node metastasis

N1 metastasis to movable homolateral axillary nodes not fixed to one another or to other structure ; further class-ified as to number of metastases and size

N2 metastasis to homolateral axillary lymph nodes that are fixed to one another or to other structures

N3 metastasis to homolateral supraclavicular or infraclavicular lymph node(s)

Distant metastases(M)

(all time periods)

MX not assessed

M0 no(known) distant metastasis

M1 distant metastasis present

specify : ____________________

Tumor size

___× ___×___ cm

Predominant lesion measured on :

patient

mammogram

pathologic specimen

Lacation (multiple when necessary)

OUQ°

OLQ°

IUQ°

ILQ°

nipple/areola

° Quadrants : outer upper, outer lower, inner upper, inner lower.

Performance status of host(H)

Several systems for recording a patient's activity and symptoms are used and are more or less equivalent as follows

H0 normal activity

H1 symptomatic but ambulatory-cares for self

H2 ambulatory more than 50% of time-occasionally needs assistance

H3 ambulatory 50% or less of time nursing care needed

H4 bedridden-may need hospitalization

Stage

clinical diagnostic

surgical evaluative

postsurgical treatment pathologic

stage TIS : in situ

stage X : cannot stage(unstageable)

stages Ⅰ-Ⅳ(further broken down ; too detailed for this text)

Histologic type of cancer (check predominant type)

Ductal

intraductal (in situ)

invasive with predominant intraductal component invasive, NOS (Not Otherwise Specified)

comedo

inflammatory

medullary with lymphocytic infiltrate

mucinous(colloid)

papillary

scirrhous

tubular

other(specify)

Lobular

in situ

invasive with predominant in situcomponent invasive

Nipple

Paget's disease, NOS

Paget's disease with intraductal carcinoma

Paget's disease with invasive ductal carcinoma other(specify)

Histologic grade

G1 : well-differentiated

G2 : moderately well-differentiated

G3-G4 : poorly to very poorly differentiated

Appendix A REVIEW SHEET

Review Sheet Number 1

Word Part	Meaning	
acr/o	______________	extremity
megal/o	______________	enlargement
dermat/o	______________	skin
cyan/o	______________	blue
derm/o	______________	skin
leuk/o	______________	white
penia	______________	lack
cardi/o	______________	heart
gastr/o	______________	stomach
cyt/o	______________	cell
algia	______________	pain
ectomy	______________	excision
tomy	______________	incision
stomy	______________	new opening
duoden/o	______________	duodenum
electr/o	______________	electricity
tome	______________	cutting instrument
emia	______________	in the blood
chlor/o	______________	green
xanth/o	______________	yellow
erythr/o	______________	red
melan/o	______________	black
thromb/o	______________	clot
blast	______________	embryonic cell
paralysis	______________	loss of movement
cheil/o	______________	lips

Review Sheet Number 2

Word Part	Meaning	
mania	______________	madness
hyper	______________	more than normal(above)
hypo	______________	less than normal(below)
emesis	______________	vomiting
throph/o	______________	development
aden/o	______________	gland
path/o	______________	disease
lip/o	______________	fat
encephal/o	______________	brain
oma	______________	tumor
cerebr/o	______________	cerebrum(brain)
crani/o	______________	cranium(skull)
mening/o	______________	meninges
carcin/o	______________	cancer
malac/o	______________	softening
muc/o	______________	mucus
cephal/o	______________	head
dynia	______________	pain
cele	______________	herniation
gram	______________	record
onych/o	______________	nail
om/o	______________	shoulder
myx/o	______________	mucus
gloss/o	______________	tongue
onych/o	______________	nail
infra	______________	under

Review Sheet Number 3

Word Part	Meaning	
ten/o	______	tendon
scope	______	looking instrument
scopy	______	looking procedure
burs/o	______	bursa(serous sac)
inter	______	between
abdomin/o	______	abdomen
hydro	______	water
phobia	______	fear
oste/o	______	bone
arthr/o	______	joint
chondr/o	______	cartilage
cost/o	______	rib
inter	______	between
dent/o	______	tooth
ab	______	from
ad	______	toward
cyst/o	______	bladder
centesis	______	puncture
thorac/o	______	thorax or chest
hydr/o	______	water
therap/o	______	treatment
pub/o	______	pubis
metero	______	uterus
pelv/i	______	pelvis
myx/o	______	mucus
supra	______	above

Review Sheet Number 4

Word Part	Meaning	
staphyl/o	______________	uvula, staphylococcus
cocc/o	______________	coccus
py/o	______________	pus
gen/o, gen/ic	______________	generation
gen/esis	______________	origin
gen/ous	______________	beginning
rrhea	______________	flow
ot/o	______________	ear
rhin/o	______________	nose
lith/o	______________	stone, calculus
chol/e	______________	bile
brad/y	______________	slow
phag/o	______________	eat
/ia		
kinesi/o	______________	movement
log/o, logy	______________	study
malac/o	______________	softening
tach/y	______________	fast
pne/o	______________	breathe
a	______________	without
dys	______________	bad, painful, difficult
peps/ia	______________	digestion
cyst/o	______________	bladder
strept/o	______________	twisted
dipl/o	______________	double
uvul/o	______________	uvula
tympan/o	______________	eardrum
ptosis	______________	prolapse

Review Sheet Number 5

Word Part	Meaning	
neur/o	______________	nerve
blast/o	______________	embryonic form
angi/o	______________	vessel
spasm	______________	spasm
scler/o	______________	hard
my/o	______________	muscle
fibr/o	______________	fibrous-fiber
lys/o	______________	destruction
lip/o	______________	fat
cyt/o	______________	cell
hem/o	______________	blood
hemat/o	______________	blood
arthr/o	______________	joint
phob/o	______________	fear
spermat/o	______________	spermatozoa
cyst/o	______________	bladder
o/o	______________	ovum
orchid/o	______________	testicle
colp/o	______________	vagina
metr/o	______________	uterus
gynec/o	______________	woman
gen/o	______________	origin, beginning
oophor/o	______________	ovary
pex/o	______________	fixation
/y		
salping/o	______________	fallopian tube
hyster/o	______________	uterus
cele	______________	herniation

Review Sheet Number 6

Word Part	Meaning	
nephr/o	______________	kidney
lith/o	______________	stone, calculus
pyel/o	______________	renal pelvis
plast/o	______________	repair
/y		
ureter/o	______________	ureter
stomy	______________	new opening
rrhaphy	______________	suture
urethr/o	______________	urethra
tomy	______________	incision
ectomy	______________	excision
cyst/o	______________	bladder
cyt/o	______________	cell
rrhagia	______________	hemorrhage
rrhea	______________	flow
pneumon/o	______________	lung
pneum/o	______________	air
pne/o	______________	breathing
melan/o	______________	black
myc/o	______________	fungus
carcin/o	______________	cancer
rhin/o	______________	nose
thorac/o	______________	thorax, chest
ur/o	______________	urine
vesic/o	______________	urinary bladder
ren/o	______________	kidney
pharmac/o	______________	drugs, medicine
ectop/o	______________	misplaced

Review Sheet Number 7

Word Part	Meaning	
stomat/o	______	mouth
dent/o	______	tooth
gloss/o	______	tongue
cheil/o	______	lip
gingiv/o	______	gum
esophag/o	______	esophagus
gastr/o	______	stomach
enter/o	______	small intestine
duoden/o	______	duodenum
col/o	______	colon
rect/o	______	rectum
proct/o	______	anus, rectum
hepat/o	______	liver
pancreat/o	______	pancreas
clys/o, clys/is	______	wash, irrigate
ectas/ia, ectas/is	______	dilatation, stretch
scop/o	______	examination
arteri/o	______	artery
pleg/a	______	paralysis
/ia		
pex/o	______	fixation
/y		
hyster/o	______	uterus
rrhea	______	flow
rrhaphy	______	suture
cyst/o	______	bladder
splen/o	______	spleen
nyct/o	______	night

Review Sheet Number 8

Word Part	Meaning	
kinesi/o	______________	movement
arteri/o	______________	artery
rrhexis	______________	rupture
rrhaphy	______________	suture
rrhea	______________	flow
rrhagia	______________	hemorrhage
esthesi/o	______________	feeling, sensation
an, a	______________	without
dys	______________	bad, painful, difficult
hypo	______________	less than normal
par/a	______________	around, beyond
hyper	______________	more than normal
alges/i	______________	abnormal sensitivity
troph/o	______________	development
lys/o	______________	destruction
oste/o	______________	bone
arthr/o	______________	joint
phas/o	______________	speech
phon/o	______________	voice
tach/y	______________	fast
brad/y	______________	slow
my/o	______________	muscle
blast/o	______________	embryonic form
fibr/o	______________	fibrous, fiber
gram/o	______________	recording
gram	______________	recorded
graph	______________	instrument
graphy	______________	process, method

Review Sheet Number 9

Word Part	Meaning	
dipl/o	______________	double
phon/o	______________	voice
opia	______________	vision
amb/i	______________	both
cocc/o	______________	coccus
cyan/o	______________	blue
neur/o	______________	nerve
tripsy	______________	surgical crushing
pyel/o	______________	renal pelvis
cyt/o	______________	cell
cyst/o	______________	bladder
cele	______________	herniation
dys	______________	bad, painful, difficult
chondr/o	______________	cartilage
cost/o	______________	rib
plas/o	______________	formation, development
psych/o	______________	mind, soul
osis	______________	condition
oma	______________	tumor
oid	______________	resembling
pro	______________	before
gnos/ia	______________	knowledge, know
di/a	______________	through
rrhea	______________	flow
rrhaphy	______________	suture
rrhagia	______________	hemorrhage
rrhexis	______________	rupture
myel/o	______________	spinal cord
pharmac/o	______________	medicine

Review Sheet Number 10

Word Part	Meaning	
therm/o	__________	heat
esthesi/o	__________	feeling
metr/o	__________	uterus
phob/o	__________	fear
pleg/a	__________	paralysis
scop/o	__________	examine
micr/o	__________	small
macr/o	__________	large
cephal/o	__________	head
myel/o	__________	bone marrow
ot/o	__________	ear
rhin/o	__________	nose
cheil/o	__________	lip
dactyl/o	__________	finger, toe
megal/o	__________	enlargement
pol/y	__________	many
ur/o	__________	urine
neur/o	__________	nerve
psych/o	__________	mind or soul
arthr/o	__________	joint
oste/o	__________	bone
syn	__________	with
drom/o	__________	running with(symptom)
ectas/ia	__________	dilatation
/is		
opia	__________	vision
than/o	__________	death
dacry/o	__________	tear

Review Sheet Number 11

Word Part	Meaning	
medi/o	____________	middle
later/o	____________	side
omphal/o	____________	umbilicus
bi/o	____________	living or life
lymph/o	____________	lymph tissue(fluid)
viscer/o	____________	organ
dips/o	____________	thirst, drink
pol/y	____________	many
mania	____________	madness
anter/o	____________	before
poster/o	____________	behind, after
dors/o	____________	back
ventr/o	____________	belly
cephal/o	____________	head
encephal/o	____________	brain
aer/o	____________	air
chrom/o	____________	color
lys/o	____________	destruction
gen/o	____________	sex
phil/o	____________	attraction
eu	____________	good
peps/ia	____________	digestion
kinesi/o	____________	movement
men/o	____________	menses, menstruation
stasis	____________	stop
syphil/o	____________	syphilis
pseud/o	____________	false
edema	____________	swelling

Review Sheet Number 12

Word Part	Meaning	
lapar/o		abdominal well
hepat/o		liver
col/o		colon
bi/o		life
pyr/o		fever, fire
xanth/o		yellow
chlor/o		green
opia		vision
erythr/o		red
leuk/o		white
melan/o		black
cyt/o		cell
cyst/o		bladder
derm/o		skin
blast/o		embryonic form
emia		blood
hidr/o		sweat
aden/o		gland
gynec/o		woman
path/o		disease
plast/o		repair
ophthalm/o		eye
viscer/o		organ
glyc/o		sugar
hypo		less than normal
later/o		side
thanato		death
enter/o		small intestine

Review Sheet Number 13

Word Part	Meaning	
mamm/o	______	breast
stern/o	______	sternum
version	______	turning
periton/o	______	peritoneum
appendic/o	______	appendix
immun/o	______	immunity
dyn/o	______	pain
spasm	______	spasm
rrhaphy	______	suture
rrhea	______	flow
rrhagia	______	hemorrhage
rrhexis	______	rupture
end/o	______	inner
mes/o	______	middle
ect/o	______	outer
hyster/o	______	uterus
ectop/o	______	misplaced
retr/o	______	behind, backward
par/a	______	around
hepat/o	______	liver
aut/o	______	self
hem/o	______	blood
py/o	______	pus
muc/o	______	mucus
opia	______	vision
ptosis	______	prolapse
sub	______	under, below
sept/o	______	infection

Review Sheet Number 14

Word Part	Meaning	
par/o	______	to bear
pyr/o	______	heat, fire
ocul/o	______	eye
or/o	______	mouth
null/i	______	none
ab	______	form
ad	______	toward
de	______	from
ex	______	from
narc/o	______	sleep
leps/y	______	seizure
is/o	______	equal
anis/o	______	unequal
dactyl/o	______	fingers, toes
peri	______	around
chondr/o	______	cartilage
cost/o	______	rib
aden/o	______	gland
circum	______	around
di/a	______	through
per	______	through
necr/o	______	dead
ectomy	______	excision
tomy	______	incision
phob/o	______	fear
phil/o	______	attraction
ectop/o	______	misplaced
phag/o	______	eat

Review Sheet Number 15

Word Part	Meaning	
pod/o	______________	foot
ren/o	______________	kidney
a or an	______________	without
meta	______________	beyond
carp/o	______________	carpals(wrist bones)
tars/o	______________	tarsals(ankle bones)
stasis	______________	control
hom/o	______________	same
heter/o	______________	different
lys/o	______________	destruction
pex/o	______________	fixation
sym	______________	together
super	______________	above
pub/o	______________	pubis
par/a	______________	bear
syn	______________	together
metr/o, hyster/o	______________	uterus
rrhexis	______________	rupture
rrhaphy	______________	suture
salping/o	______________	fallopian tube
oophor/o	______________	ovary
epi	______________	over, upon
extra	______________	beyond, outside
phag/o	______________	eat
anti	______________	against
contra	______________	against
trans	______________	across
trips/y	______________	crushing

Review Sheet Number 16

Word Part	Meaning	
sept/o	______	infection
phag/o	______	eat
anti	______	against
contra	______	against
trans	______	across
trips/y	______	crushing
ectop/o	______	misplaced
vagin/o	______	vagina
urethr/o	______	urethra
in	______	in, not
somn/i	______	sleep
cis/e	______	cut
mal	______	bad
sanguin/o	______	blood
natal	______	birth
febrile	______	fever
partum	______	birth
tri	______	three
bi	______	two, double
semi	______	half
hemi	______	half
troph/o	______	development
con	______	with
dis	______	separation
post	______	after, behind
pre	______	before, in front of
intra	______	within
fung/i	______	fungus

Review Sheet Number 17

Word Part	Meaning	
phren/o		diaphragm
stomy		permanent opening
lith/o		stone
pleur/o		pleural membrane
plegia		paralysis
ped/o		foot
man/o		hand
pod/o		foot
chir/o		hand
hist/o		tissue
cervic/o		neck of uterus, neck
nas/o		nose
pharyng/o		pharynx
laryng/o		larynx
trache/o		trachea
bronch/o		bronchus
pleur/o		pleura
centesis		puncture
sinistr/o		left
dextr/o		right
vas/o		vessel
ne/o		new
penia		lack of
splen/o		spleen
infra		below, under
sub		under, below
sept/o		infection
omphal/o		navel

Review Sheet Number 18

Word Part	Meaning	
noct/i, nyct/o	____________	night
opia	____________	vision
ankyl/o	____________	stiff
phor/o	____________	bear, carry
eu	____________	good, well, easy
stasis	____________	stopping, controlling
calcane/o	____________	heel
carp/o	____________	wrist
schiz/o, schist/o	____________	split
ischi/o	____________	ischium
stern/o	____________	sterum
phalang/o	____________	phalanges
acromi/o	____________	acromion
humer/o	____________	humerus
condyl/o	____________	condyle
gangli/o	____________	ganglia
thromb/o	____________	clot, thrombus
trich/o	____________	hair
rrhexis	____________	rupture
ectop/o	____________	misplaced
ante	____________	before, forward
plasm/o	____________	formation
lumb/o	____________	lumbar
uln/o	____________	ulnar
radi/o	____________	radius
scapul/o	____________	scapula
phren/o	____________	mind, diaphragm
enter/o	____________	small intestine

Review Sheet Number 19

Word Part	Meaning	
ophthalm/o	______	eye
xanth/o	______	yellow
chlor/o	______	green
erythr/o	______	red
blephar/o	______	eyelid
py/o	______	pus
phag/o	______	ingesting
trich/o	______	hair
traumat/o	______	injury
onc/o	______	neoplasms
corne/o	______	cornea
scler/o	______	sclera
ir/o, irid/o	______	iris
retin/o	______	retina
cor/e, core/o	______	pupil
kerat/o	______	cornea
cycl/o	______	ciliary body
pleg/ia	______	paralysis
lacrim/o, dacry/o	______	tear
tome	______	instrument for incising
tympan/o	______	eardrum
ren/o	______	kidney
vesic/o	______	bladder
pod/o	______	foot
chir/o	______	hands
crypt/o	______	hidden
emia	______	blood
rachi/o, rach/i	______	spine

Review Sheet Number 20

Count using these prefixes.

Prefix	Meaning	
mono	______________	single, one
multi	______________	many
nulli	______________	none
primi	______________	first
uni	______________	one
bi	______________	two
diplo	______________	double
tri	______________	three
quadri, tetra	______________	four
quinque, penta	______________	five
hex, sex	______________	six
septa, hepta	______________	seven
octa	______________	eight
nona	______________	nine
deca	______________	ten
hecto	______________	one hundred
kilo	______________	one thousand
deci	______________	one tenth
centi	______________	one hundredth
milli	______________	one thousanth
micro	______________	one millionth
nano	______________	one billionth

Review Sheet Number 21

Make plurals of these simgular terms.

Singular	Piural	
bursa	______	bursae
conjunctiva	______	conjunctivae
fossa	______	fossae
vertebra	______	vertebrae
pleura	______	pleurae
cornea	______	corneae
bacillus	______	bacilli
bronchus	______	bronchi
coccus	______	cocci
focus	______	foci
locus	______	loci
nucleus	______	nuclei
atrium	______	atria
ileum	______	ilea
bacterium	______	bacteria
carcinoma	______	carcinomata
lipoma	______	lipomata
condyloma	______	condylomata
enema	______	enemata
ganglion	______	ganglia
spermatozoon	______	spermatozoa
diagnosis	______	diagnoses
pelvis	______	pelves
appendix	______	appendices
thorax	______	thoraces
cervix	______	cervices

Review Sheet Number 22

Meaning	Word Part	
double	______	diplo
many	______	multi
five	______	penta
seven	______	hepta
one hundred	______	hecto
eight	______	octa
two	______	bi
nine	______	nona
ten	______	deca
single/one	______	mono
first	______	primi
one thousand	______	kilo
four	______	quadri
six	______	hexa
none	______	nulli
one	______	uni
three	______	tri
one tenth	______	deci
one hundredth	______	centi
one thousandth	______	milli
one millionth	______	micro
one billionth	______	nano

Review Sheet Number 23

Meaning	Word Part	
tumor	______	oma
cerebrum(brain)	______	cerebr/o
cranium(skull)	______	crani/o
meninges	______	mening/o
cancer	______	carcin/o
softening	______	malac/o
mucus	______	muc/o
head	______	cephal/o
pain	______	dynia
record	______	gram
brain	______	encephal/o
fat	______	lip/o
disease	______	path/o
gland	______	aden/o
development	______	throph/o
vomiting	______	emesis
less than normal(below)	______	hypo
more than normal(above)	______	hyper
madness	______	mania
herniation	______	cele
artery	______	arteri/o
movement	______	kinesi/o
hemorrhage	______	orrhagia
vein	______	phleb/o
around(beyond)	______	par/a

Review Sheet Number 24

Meaning	Word Part	
thorax, chest	______________	thorac/o
puncture	______________	centesis
bladder	______________	cyst/o
abdomen	______________	abdomin/o
toward	______________	ad
from	______________	ab
tooth	______________	dent/o
between	______________	inter
rib	______________	cost/o
cartilage	______________	chondr/o
joint	______________	arthr/o
bone	______________	oste/o
pelvis	______________	pelv/i
water	______________	hydr/o
treatment	______________	therap/o
pubis	______________	pub/o
measure	______________	metr/o, meter
fear	______________	phobia
fast	______________	tach/y
slow	______________	brad/y
between	______________	inter
bursa(serous sac)	______________	burs/o
looking procedure	______________	scopy
looking instrument	______________	scope
tendon	______________	ten/o

Review Sheet Number 25

Meaning	Word Part	
uvula	______________	uvul/o
eardrum	______________	tympan/o
double	______________	dipl/o
flow	______________	orrhea
slow	______________	brad/y
digestion	______________	peps/ia
twisted	______________	strept/o
gall-bile	______________	chol/e
nose	______________	rhin/o
pus	______________	py/o
movement	______________	kinesi/o
fast	______________	tach/y
beginning	______________	gen/ous, gen/o
breathe	______________	pne/o
bladder	______________	cyst/o
bad, painful, difficult	______________	dys
coccus	______________	cocc/o
without	______________	a
study	______________	log/o, logy
stone, calculus	______________	lith/o
eat	______________	phag/o
uvula, staphylococcus	______________	staphyl/o
ear	______________	ot/o
softening	______________	malac/o
fat	______________	lip/o

REVIEW SHEET Number 26

Meaning	Word Part	
woman	______	gynec/o
vagina	______	colp/o
metr/o	______	uterine tissues
testicle	______	orchid/o
fear	______	phob/o
vessel	______	angi/o
uterus	______	hyster/o
destruction	______	lys/o
origin, beginning	______	gen/o
prolapse	______	ptosis
blood	______	hem/o, hemat/o
bladder	______	cyst/o
hard	______	scler/o
joint	______	arthr/o
fallopian tube	______	salping/o
muscle	______	my/o
nerve	______	neur/o
fixation	______	pex/o
ovum	______	o/o
cell	______	cyt/o
embryonic form	______	blast/o
ovary	______	oophor/o
herniation	______	cele
disease	______	path/o
spermatozoa	______	spermat/o

Review Sheet Number 27

Meaning	Word Part	
hemorrhage	______________	orrhagia
cell	______________	cyt/o
renal pelvis	______________	pyel/o
measure	______________	meter, metr/o
urine	______________	ur/o
kidney	______________	ren/o
urinary bladder	______________	vesic/o
black	______________	melan/o
ureter	______________	ureter/o
excision	______________	ectomy
kidney	______________	nephr/o
cancer	______________	carcin/o
lung	______________	pneumon/o
urethra	______________	urethr/o
thorax, chest	______________	thorac/o
air	______________	pneum/o
suture	______________	orrhaphy
nose	______________	rhin/o
fungus	______________	myc/o
breathing	______________	pne/o
flow	______________	orrhea
bladder	______________	cyst/o
incision	______________	otomy
new opening	______________	ostomy
repair	______________	plast/o

Review Sheet Number 28

Meaning	Word Part	
paralysis		pleg/a
stomach		gastr/o
rectum		rect/o
duodenum		duoden/o
liver		hepat/o
suture		orrhaphy
small intestine		enter/o
spleen		splen/o
tooth		dent/o
flow		orrhea
artery		arteri/o
anus, rectum		proct/o
lip		cheil/o
wash-irrigate		clys/is, clys/o
esophagus		esophag/o
uterus		hyster/o
bladder		cyst/o
fixation		pex/o
pancreas		pancreat/o
examination		scop/o
colon		col/o
gum		gingiv/o
mouth		stomat/o
dilatation-stretch		ectas/ia
tongue		gloss/o

Review Sheet Number 29

Meaning	Word Part	
destruction	______	lys/o
fast	______	tach/y
flow	______	orrhea
more than normal	______	hyper
fibrous, fiber	______	fibr/o
without	______	an, a
bone	______	oste/o
joint	______	arthr/o
recording	______	gram/o
the process	______	graphy
the instrument	______	graph
the record	______	gram
bad, painful, difficult	______	dys
rupture	______	orrhexis
voice	______	phon/o
muscle	______	my/o
feeling, sensation	______	esthesi/o
less than normal	______	hypo
development	______	troph/o
embryonic form	______	blast/o
slow	______	brad/y
suture	______	orrhaphy
abnormal sensitivity	______	alges/i
study	______	log/o
speech	______	phas/o

Review Sheet Number 30

Meaning	Word Part	
drugs, medicine	______	pharmac/o
spinal cord	______	myel/o
cell	______	cyt/o
formation, development	______	plas/o
double	______	dipl/o
tumor	______	oma
flow	______	orrhea
blue	______	cyan/o
herniation	______	cele
condition	______	osis
rupture	______	orrhexis
coccus	______	cocc/o
renal pelvis	______	pyel/o
mind, soul	______	psych/o
through	______	di/a
rib	______	cost/o
hemorrhage	______	orrhagia
voice	______	phon/o
surgical crushing	______	trips/y
suture	______	orrhaphy
resembling	______	oid
both	______	amb/i
carilage	______	chondr/o
before	______	pro
stone	______	lith/o

Review Sheet Number 31

Meaning	Word Part	
bone marrow	______________	myel/o
measure	______________	metr/o, meter
mind, soul	______________	psych/o
nose	______________	rhin/o
paralysis	______________	pleg/ia
large	______________	macr/o
with	______________	syn
heat	______________	therm/o
finger, toe	______________	dactyl/o
urine	______________	ur/o
examine	______________	scop/o
symptom	______________	drom/o
enlargement	______________	megal/o
bone	______________	oste/o
many	______________	pol/y
ear	______________	ot/o
joint	______________	arthr/o
feeling	______________	esthesi/o
small	______________	micr/o
nerve	______________	neur/o
lip	______________	cheil/o
head	______________	cephal/o
fear	______________	phob/o
dilatation	______________	ectas/ia
nerve	______________	neur/o

Review Sheet Number 32

Meaning	Word Part	
back	______________	dors/o
attraction	______________	phil/o
vision	______________	opia
madness	______________	mania
destruction	______________	lys/o
menses, menstruation	______________	men/o
swelling	______________	edema
measure	______________	metr/o, meter
thirst, drink	______________	dips/o
death	______________	than/o
middle	______________	medi/o
organ	______________	viscer/o
side	______________	later/o
lymph tissue(fluid)	______________	lymph/o
living, life	______________	bi/o
umbilicus	______________	omphal/o
small intestine	______________	enter/o
brain	______________	encephal/o
digestion	______________	peps/ia
syphilis	______________	syphil/o
prolapse	______________	ptosis
air	______________	aer/o
belly	______________	ventro/o
before	______________	anter/o
vision	______________	opia

Review Sheet Number 33

Meaning	Word Part	
gland	______________	aden/o
skin	______________	derm/o
white	______________	leuk/o
yellow	______________	xanth/o
disease	______________	path/o
bladder	______________	cyst/o
side	______________	later/o
organ	______________	viscer/o
sweat	______________	hidr/o
abdominal wall	______________	lapar/o
eye	______________	ophthalm/o
fever, fire	______________	pyr/o
less than normal	______________	hypo
embryonic form	______________	blast/o
liver	______________	hepat/o
woman	______________	gynec/o
black	______________	melan/o
sugar	______________	glyc/o
life	______________	bi/o
red	______________	erythr/o
blood	______________	emia
repair	______________	plast/o
colon	______________	col/o
green	______________	chor/o
vision	______________	opia

Review Sheet Number 34

Meaning	Word Part	
outer, outside	______________	ect/o
pain	______________	dyn/o
rupture	______________	orrhexis
breast	______________	mamm/o
sternum	______________	stern/o
inner	______________	end/o
mucus	______________	muc/o
flow	______________	orrhea
behind, backward	______________	retr/o
turning	______________	version
peritoneum	______________	periton/o
blood	______________	hem/o
appendix	______________	appendic/o
middle	______________	mes/o
suture	______________	orrhaphy
immunity	______________	immun/o
uterus	______________	hyster/o
around	______________	par/a
pus	______________	py/o
liver	______________	hepat/o
misplaced	______________	ectop/o
hemorrhage	______________	orrhagia
bladder	______________	cyst/o
bad, painful	______________	dys
knowledge	______________	gnos/ia

Review Sheet Number 35

Meaning	Word Part	
cartilage	______________	chondr/o
sleep	______________	narc/o
fingers, toes	______________	dactyl/o
attraction	______________	phil/o
from	______________	de, ab, ex
many	______________	pol/y
false	______________	pseud/o
heat, fire	______________	pyr/o
mouth	______________	or/o
eye	______________	ocul/o
to bear	______________	par/o
incision	______________	otomy
rib	______________	cost/o
toward	______________	ad
excision	______________	ectomy
fear	______________	phob/o
none	______________	null/i
seizure	______________	leps/y
dead	______________	necr/o
equal	______________	is/o
gland	______________	aden/o
through	______________	per, di/a
head	______________	cephal/o
misplaced	______________	ectop/o
color	______________	chrom/o

Review Sheet Number 36

Meaning	Word Part	
tarsals(ankle bones)	______________	tars/o
carpals(wrist bones)	______________	carp/o
good	______________	eu
without	______________	a, an
kidney	______________	ren/o
foot	______________	pod/o
under, below	______________	sub
below, under	______________	infra
in addition to, beyond	______________	extra
over, upon	______________	epi
ovary	______________	oophor/o
fallopian tube	______________	salping/o
suture	______________	orrhaphy
rupture	______________	orrhexis
uterus	______________	metr/o, hyster/o
together	______________	syn
bear	______________	par/a
above	______________	supra
pubis	______________	pub/o
sleep	______________	somn/i
together	______________	sym
fixation	______________	pex/o
destruction	______________	lys/o
different	______________	heter/o
same	______________	hom/o

Review Sheet Number 37

Meaning	Word Part	
within	______________	intra
before, in front of	______________	pre
after, behind	______________	post
to free, to undo	______________	dis
with	______________	con
development	______________	troph/o
half	______________	hemi, semi
unequal	______________	anis/o
two, double	______________	bi
three	______________	tri
cut	______________	cis/e
sleep	______________	somn/i
green	______________	chlor/o
urethra	______________	urethr/o
vagina	______________	vagin/o
birth	______________	partum
fever	______________	febrile
birth	______________	natal
blood	______________	sanguin/o
bad	______________	mal
misplaced	______________	ectop/o
crushing	______________	trips/y
across, over	______________	trans
against	______________	contra
behind	______________	poster/o

Review Sheet Number 38

Meaning	Word Part	
nose	______________	nas/o
pleura	______________	pleur/o
before, in front of	______________	pre
lack of	______________	penia
one	______________	uni
larynx	______________	laryng/o
puncture	______________	centesis
right	______________	dextr/o
bronchus	______________	bronch/o
vessel	______________	vas/o
spleen	______________	splen/o
three	______________	tri
left	______________	sinistr/o
trachea	______________	trache/o
new	______________	ne/o
pharynx	______________	pharyng/o
neck of uterus, neck	______________	cervic/o
tissue	______________	hist/o
hand	______________	chir/o
foot	______________	pod/o, ped/o
hand	______________	man/o
eat	______________	phag/o
paralysis	______________	pleg/ia
pleural membrane	______________	pleur/o
against	______________	anti

Review Sheet Number 39

Meaning	Word Part	
lips	______	cheil/o
tongue	______	gloss/o
fungus	______	fung/i, myc/o
small intestine	______	enter/o
mind, diaphragm	______	phren/o
scapula	______	scapul/o
radius	______	radi/o
ulnar	______	uln/o
lumbar	______	lumb/o
spine	______	rachi/o, rach/i
split	______	schisis, schist/o,
infection	______	sept/o, seps/is
bear, carry	______	phor/o
night	______	nyct/o, noct/i
diaphragm	______	phren/o
before, forward	______	ante
wrist	______	carp/o
formation	______	plasm/o, plas/o, troph/o,
permanent opening	______	ostomy
clot, thrombus	______	thromb/o
stopping, controlling	______	stasis
hair	______	trich/o
humerus	______	humer/o
heel	______	calcane/o
vision	______	opia

Review Sheet Number 40

Meaning	Word Part	
bladder	__________	vesic/o
misplaced	__________	ectop/o
cornea	__________	corne/o, kerat/o
blood	__________	emia
mucus	__________	myx/o, muc/o
instrument for incising	__________	tome
iris	__________	ir/o, irid/o
movement	__________	kinesi/o
diaphragm	__________	phren/o
retina	__________	retin/o
tear	__________	dacry/o, lacrim/o
around	__________	peri, circum
nail	__________	onych/o
hands	__________	chir/o
eardrum	__________	tympan/o
shoulder	__________	om/o
navel	__________	omphal/o
ciliary body	__________	cycl/o
sclera	__________	scler/o
foot	__________	pod/o
neoplasms	__________	onc/o
injury	__________	traumat/o
hair	__________	trich/o
ingesting	__________	phag/o
repture	__________	orrhexis

Review Sheet Number 41

Meaning	Word Part	
cutting instrument	______________	tome
in the blood	______________	emia
green	______________	chlor/o
enlargement	______________	megal/o
electricity	______________	electr/o
white	______________	leuk/o
yellow	______________	xanth/o
incision	______________	otomy
blue	______________	cyan/o
red	______________	erythr/o
stomach	______________	gastr/o
extremity	______________	acr/o
black	______________	melan/o
new opening	______________	ostomy
color	______________	chrom/o
heart	______________	cardi/o
skin	______________	derm/o, dermat/o
clot	______________	thromb/o
embryonic cell	______________	blast
excision	______________	ectomy
lack of	______________	penia
duodenum	______________	duoden/o
pain	______________	algia
cell	______________	cyt/o
loss of movement	______________	paralysis

Review Sheet Number 42

Meaning	Word Part	
pus	______________	py/o
eyelid	______________	blephar/o
red	______________	erythr/o
green	______________	chlor/o
yellow	______________	xanth/o
eye	______________	ophthalm/o
spine	______________	rachi/o, rach/i
hidden	______________	crypt/o
kidney	______________	ren/o
pupil	______________	cor/e, core/o
paralysis	______________	pleg/ia
heel	______________	calcane/o
misplaced	______________	ectop/o
sternum	______________	stern/o
rupture	______________	orrhexis
ganglia	______________	gangli/o
ischium	______________	ischi/o
vision	______________	opia
condyle	______________	condyl/o
acromion	______________	acromi/o
good, well, easy	______________	eu
phalanges	______________	phalang/o
stiff	______________	ankyl/o
control	______________	stasis
fixation	______________	pex/o

Appendix B ABBREVIATIONS

Abbreviations Number 1

WEIGHTS AND MEASURES		
Metric		
kg	kilogram(s) (1000 g)	
hg	hectogram (100 g)	
dag	decagram (10 g)	
g or gm	gram	
dg	decigram (0.1 g)	
cg	centigram (0.01 g)	
mg	milligram (0.001 g)	
μg or mcg	microgram (0.001 mg)	
Standard		
lb, #	pound	
oz, symbol	ounce	
dr, symbol	dram	
gr	grain	
Volume		
cumm	cubic millimeter (mm^3)	
cc	cubic centimeter (cm^3)	
cum	cubic meter (m^3)	
cu in	cubic inch (in^3)	
cu ft	cubic foot (ft^3)	
cu yd	cubic yard (yd^3)	
Lengths		
in, "	inch (2.54 cm)	
ft, '	foot (12 in)	
yd	yard (36 in)	
mm	millimeter (0.001 m)	
cm	centimeter (0.01 m)	
m	meter	
km	kilometer (1000 m)	

Abbreviations Number 2

WEIGHTS AND MEASURES		
Liquid Volume		
t, tsp	teaspoon	
T, Tbsp	tablespoon	
c	cup	
m, min	minims	
ml	milliliter (0.001 L)	
cc	cubic centimeter (1 ml)	
cl	centiliter (0.01 L)	
dl	deciliter (0.1 L)	
L	liter (1000 ml)	
dal	decaliter (10 L)	
hl	hectoliter (100 L)	
kl	kiloliter (1000 L)	
fl dr	fluid dram (60 min)	
fl oz	fluid ounce (8 fl dr)	
pt	pint (16 oz)	
qt	quart (32 oz)	
gal	gallon (4 qt)	
gt	drop (1 min)	
gtt	drops	
Miscellaneous		
at wt	atomic weight	
C, kcal	calorie	
c	curie	
ht	height	
mA	milliampere	
mEq	milliequivalent	
mHz	megahertz	
mg%	milligram percent	
mw	molecular weight	
IU	international units	
U	units	

Appendix B

Abbreviations Number 3

CHEMICAL		
Symbols		
Al	aluminum	____________
Ar	argon	____________
As	arsenic	____________
Ba	barium	____________
B	boron	____________
Br	bromine	____________
Cd	cadmium	____________
Ca	calcium [Ca^{2+} ion]	____________
C	carbon	____________
CO_2	carbon dioxide	____________
Cl	chlorine [Cl^- ion]	____________
Cr	chromium	____________
Co	cobalt	____________
Cu	copper [Cu^{2+} ion]	____________
F	fluorine	____________
$C_6H_{12}O_6$	glucose	____________
He	helium	____________
H	hydrogen	____________
I	iodine [^{131}I radioactive]	____________
Fe	iron	____________
Kr	krypton	____________
Pb	lead	____________
Li	lithium	____________
Mg	magnesium	____________
Mn	manganese	____________
Hg	mercury	____________
Ne	neon	____________
N	nitrogen	____________
O	oxygen (O_2)	____________
P	phosphorus	____________
K	potassium	____________
Ra	radium	____________
Se	selenium	____________
Si	silicon	____________
Ag	silver	____________
$AgNO_3$	silver nitrate	____________
Na	sodium	____________
NaCl	sodium chloride	____________
S	sulfur	____________
U	uranium	____________
Zn	zinc	____________

Abbreviations Number 4

DIAGNOSES		
ABE	acute bacterial endocarditis	
ACVD	acute cardiovascular disease	
AF (Afib)	artial fibrillation	
AI	aortic insufficiency	
AID	acute infectious disease	
	artificial insemination donor	
AIDS	acquired immune deficiency syndrome	
AIH	artificial insemination husband	
ALL	acute lymphocytic leukemia	
ALS	amyotrophic lateral scoliosis	
AMI	acute myocardial infarction	
AOD	arterial occlusive disease	
ARC	AIDS Related Complex (Conditions)	
ARD	acute respiratory disease	
ARF	acute respiratory failure	
	acute renal failure	
ARV	acute rheumatic fever	
AS	AIDS Related Virus	
	aortic stenosis	
	arteriosclerosis	
ASCVD	left ear(auris sinistra)	
ASHD	arteriosclerotic cardiovascular disease	
BCC	arteriosclerotic heart disease	
BO	basal cell carcinoma	
Ca	body odor	
CAD	cancer	
CHD	coronary artery disease	
	congestive heart disease	
	congenital hip dislocation	
CE	cardiac enlargement	
CF	cystic fibrosis	
CHD	congenital or coronary heart disease	
	childhood disease	
CHF	congestive heart failure	
CIS	carcinoma in situ	
CLD	chronic liver disease	
	chronic lung disease	

Abbreviations Number 5

DIAGNOSES		
COLD	chronic obstructive lung disease	
COPD	chronic obstructive pulmonary disease	
CP	cerebral palsey	
CPD	cephalopelvic disproportion	
CRF	chronic renal failure	
CT	carpal tunnel	
	coronary thrombosis	
CVA	cerebrovascular accident	
CVD	cardiovascular disease	
DOA	dead on arrival	
DRG	Diagnostic Related Groups	
DTs	delirim tremens	
Dx	diagnosis	
ESRD	end-stage renal failure	
FB	foreign body	
FOD	free of disease	
FTND	full-trem normal delivery	
FTT	failure to thrive	
FUO	fever of unknown origin	
Fx	fracture	
FxBB	fracture both bones	
GNID	gram-negativ intracellular diplococci	
Grav 1/ab 1	one pregnancy/one abortion	
HA	headache	
	hearing aid	
	hemolytic anemia	
HAA	hepatitis-associated antigen	
HC	Huntington's chorea	
HCVD	hypertensive cardiovascular disease	
HD	Hodgkin's disease	
HDN	hemolytic disease of newborn	
HF	heart failure	
HH	hiatal hernia	
HLV	herpes-like virus	
HSV	herpes simplex virus	
HTLV-III/LAV	Human T-cell lymphotropic virus III/ Lymphadenopathy associated virus	

Appendix B

Abbreviations Number 6

DIAGNOSES		
IHD	ischemic heart disease	
IM	infectious mononucleosis	
JOB	juvenile-onset diabetes	
LE	lupus erythematosus	
LGB	Landry-Guillan-Barré syndrome	
MBD	minimal brain dysfunction	
MD	manic depressive	
	muscular dystrophy	
	myocardial disease	
met, metas	metastases	
MVP	mitral valve prolapse	
MOD	maturity onset diabetes	
Mono	mononucleosis	
MS	mitral stenosis	
	multiple sclerosis	
OA	osteoarthritis	
OAG	open-angle glaucoma	
OM	otitis media	
PAR	perennial allergic rhinitis	
para	paraplegic	
para(I, II)	one live birth (two...)	
PCD	polycystic disease	
PD	Parkinson's disease	
	pulmonary disease	
PKU	phenylketonuria	
PND	paroxysmal nocturnal dyspnea	
preg	pregnant	
PVC	premature ventricular contraction	
PE	pulmonary edema	
S-C disease	sickle cell hemoglobin-c disease	
schiz	schizophrenia	
SIDS	sudden infant death syndrome	
TB	tuberculosis, tuberculin bacillus	
Thal	thalassemia	
TIA	transischemic attack	
TSD	Tay-Sachs disease	
URI	upper respiratory disease	
UTI	urinary tract infection	

Abbreviations Number 7

PROCEDURES		
AB	abrotion	______
A+P	auscultation and percussion	______
ABO	blood typing groups	______
ACTH	adrenocortiotropic hormone (test)	______
AFB	acid-fast bacillus	______
ANA	antinuclear antibodies	______
BE, BaE	barium enema	______
BCG	immunization, B-scan sonogram	______
BP	blood pressure	______
BUN	blood urea nitrogen	______
Bx, BI	biopsy	______
CAB	coronary artery bypass	______
CAD	computer-aided design	______
CBC	complete blood count	______
CAPD	chronic ambulatory peritoneal dialysis	______
Ch, Chol	cholesterol	______
CPK	creatine phosphokinase	______
CPR	cardiopulmonary resuscitation	______
C+S	culture and sensitivity	______
C section	Cesarean section	______
CT	computed tomography	______
CXR	chest x-rey	______
Cysto	cystoscopy	______
CPAP	continuous positive airway pressure ventilation	______
CSF	cerebrospinal fluid	______
D & C	dilation and curettage	______
Del	delivery	______
DHT	dihydrotestosterone	______
DNA	deoxyribonucleic acid	______
DPT	diphtheria pertussis	______
ECG, EKG	electrocardiogram	______
ECHO	echocardiogram	______
ECT	electroconvulsive therapy	______
EEG	electroencephalogram	______
EMIT	enzyme immunoassay for drug screening	______
EMG	electromyogram	______
ERG	electroretinogram	______

Appendix B

Abbreviations Number 8

PROCEDURES		
ex	excise	
exam	examination	
FBS	fasting blood sugar	
FME	full mouth extraction	
FSH	follicle stimulating hormone	
GA	gastric analysis	
GT, GTT	glucose tolerance test	
GxT	graded exercise test	
HAA	hepatitis Australian antigen	
HAI	hemagglutination inhibitionrubella test	
Hb, Hgb	hemoglobin	
Hct	hematocrit	
HDL	high density lipoproteins	
H+P	history and physical	
HGH	human growth hormone	
HSG	hysterosalpingogram	
Hx	history	
IABP	intra-aortic balloon pump	
ICSH	interstitial cell stimulating hormone	
ICAT	indirect Coomb's test	
I+D	incision and drainage	
IPPB	intermittent positive-pressure breathing	
IVP	intravenous pyelogram	
KUB	kidney ureter bladder(x-ray)	
lab	laboratory	
LASER	light amplification by stimulated emission of radiation	
LDH	lactose dehydrogenase	
LP	lumbar puncture	
LH	luteinizing hormone	
LOS	length of stay	
MASER	microwave amplification by stimulated emission of radiation	
MMRV	measles, mumps, rubella vaccine	
OC	office call	
O+P	ova and parasites test	
OPG	oculoplethysmography	

Abbreviations Number 9

PROCEDURES		
P+A	percussion and auscultation	
Pap	Papanicolaou test	
PBI	protein bound iodine	
PCV	packed cell volume	
PE	physical exam	
pH	hydrogen ion concentration, acid/base	
Pt, protime	prothrombin time	
PTT	partial thromboplastin time	
2hr pc	2-hour postcibal blood glucose	
2hr pg	2-hour postglucose blood glucose	
2hr pp	2-hour postprandial blood glucose	
P+V	pyloroplasty and vagotomy	
RIA	radioimmunoassay	
RPR	syphills test (also : ART, VDRL, STS)	
RATx	radiation therapy	
Rx	take, prescribe	
RPG	retrograde pyelogram	
SGOT	serum glutamic oxaloacetic transaminase	
SGPT	serum glutamic pyruvic transminase	
SOP	standard operating procedure	
Sp gr	specific gravity (urine)	
T_3, T_4	thyroid test	
T	temperature	
TSH	thyroid stimulating hormone	
TAA	total abdominal hysterectomy	
TENS	transcutaneous electrical nerve stimulation	
TUR	transurethral resection	
Tx	treatment	
XM	cross-match for blood	
XR	x-ray	
VCG	vectocardiogram	
VDRL	syphilis test	
YAG	yttrium aluminum garnet(laser)	
V, Y, W, Z, -plasty	various types of procedures used to repair lacerations	

Abbreviations Number 10

HEALTH PROFESSIONS		
AAMA	American Association of Medical Assistants	________
AMA	American Medical Association	________
AOA	American Osteopathic Association	________
ASCP	American Society of clinical Pathology	________
CMA	Certified Medical Assistant	________
CPHA	Commission on Professional and Hospital Activities	________
DDS	Doctor of Dental Surgery	________
DC	Doctor of Chiropractic	________
DO	Doctor of Osteopathy	________
DPM	Doctor of Podiatric Medicine	________
EENT	Eye, Ear, Nose, and Throat specialist	________
EMT	Emergency Medical Technician	________
ENT	Ear, Nose, and Throat specialist	________
FACP	Fellow of the American College of Physicians	________
FACS	Fellow of the American College of Surgeons	________
GYN	gynecology	________
LPN	Licensed practical Nurse	________
LVN	Licensed Vocational Nurse	________
MD	medical doctor	________
MT	medical technologist	________
NP	nurse practitioner	________
ORTH	orthopedist	________
OB	obstetrician	________
OT	occupational therapist	________
PA	physician's assistant	________
PC	professional corporation	________
PT	physical therapy	________
RRA	Registered Records Administrator	________
RRT	registered Radiography Technician	________
RT	respiratory therapist	________

Abbreviations Number 11

CHARTING ABBREVIATIONS		
aa	of each	
ac	before meals	
ad	right ear (auricle dexter)	
aj	ankle jerk	
adm	admission	
ant	anterior	
am	mornings	
approx	approximately	
AP	anteroposterior	
AV	atrioventricular	
ax	axillary	
bid	twice a day (bis in die)	
bin	twice a night (bis in noctus)	
BMR	basal metabolism rate	
BM	bowel movement	
BP	blood pressure	
$\overline{c}$, /w	with	
C1, C2, C3, ···	cervical vertebra first, second, third, ···	
C	centigrade	
cap(s)	capsules	
CC	chief complaint	
CCU	cardiac care unit	
c/o	complains of	
cont	continue	
D	diopter (ocular measure)	
dc	discontinue	
DC	discharge from hospital	
Dr	doctor	
Dx	diagnosis	
DNA	does not apply	
DNS	did not show	
EOM	extraocular movements	
Ex	examination	
F	Fahrenheit	
fhs	fetal heart sounds	
fht	fetal heart tones	
GB	gall bladder	
GI	gastrointestinal	
GU	genitourinary	
hpf	high power field	
hs	hour of sleep, bedtime (hora somni)	

Appendix B

Abbreviations Number 12

CHARTING ABBREVIATIONS		
hypo	hypodermically	
ICU	intensive care unit	
IM	intramuscular	
I+O	intake and output	
iss	one and one half	
IV	intravenous	
L	left	
L1, L2, L3, ···	lumbar vertebrae first, second, third, ···	
L+A	light and accommodation	
L+W	living and well	
lmp	last menstrual period	
lpf	low-power field(10×)	
LUQ	left upper quadrant of abdomen	
MTD	right eardrum (membrana tympani dexter)	
MTS	left eardrum (membrana tympani sinister)	
NPO	nothing by mouth	
neg	negative	
OD	right eye (oculus dexter)	
OLA	occipital lay anterior(fetal presentation)	
OP	outpatient	
OS	left eye (oculus sinister)	
OU	both eyes (oculus uterque)	
P	pulse	
PA	posteroanterior	
pc	after meals (post cibum)	
PDR	Physician's Desk Reference	
PI	present illness	
po	by mouth, postoperative	
pm	afternoon or evening	
prn	as needed or desired (pro re nata)	
q	every (quaque)	
qh	every hour	
q2h	every two hours	
qid	four times a day (quarter in die)	
qm	every morning	
qn	every night	
R	right, respiration	
RBC	red blood cell, erythrocyte	

Appendix B

Abbreviations Number 13

CHARTING ABBREVIATIONS		
Rh	blood factor, Rh^+ or Rh^-	
RLQ	right lower quadrant(abdomen)	
RO, R/O	rule out	
RUQ	right upper quadrant(abdomen)	
$\bar{s}$, w/o	without (sans)	
sc, subcu	subcutaneously(into fat layer)	
sed rate	sedimentation rate(blood)	
SOB	short of breath	
ss	half	
staph	staphylococcus	
stat	immediately(statum)	
strep	streptococcus	
T_1, T_2, T_3, ...	thoracic vertebrae first, second, third, ...	
T	temperature	
tab(s)	tablets	
tid	three times a day	
tinct	tincture	
ULQ	upper left quadrant (abdomen)	
ung	ointment (unguentum)	
URQ	upper right quadrant (abdomen)	
WBC	white blood cell, leukocyte count	
WM, BM	white male, black male	
WF, BF	white female, black female	
x	times, power	
y/o, yrs	years old	
+	positive	
—	negative	
♀	female	
♂	male	
+/—	positive or negative	
$\bar{p}$	after	
$\bar{a}$	before	
↑	increase	
↓	decrease	
>	greater than	
<	less than	

Appendix B

Medical Terminology

정가 25,000원

ISBN 978-89-7043-643-2

2008년 6월 20일 1판 인 쇄
2008년 6월 25일 1판 발 행

저 자 : 신영순 · 김대식 · 김봉경 · 김양호
박상묵 · 박창은 · 심문정 · 육근돌
이영종 · 이재식 · 허성호 · 현성희
최원창 · 황구연 · 홍승복 · 최승구

발 행 자 : 최 병 진

발 행 처 : 도서출판 **고 려 의 학**

(110-524) 서울시 종로구 명륜4가 91
Tel. 765-0333 / 0337
Fax. 743-2288

등록번호 : 제 1-519호 1978. 6. 29.